T0157203

kundalini
yoga massage

kundalini yoga massage

SEVEN STEPS
TO ACTIVATE THE
SEVEN
CHAKRAS
AND POWER PEOPLE'S
PRANA

DR. GITA KALIPERSHAD-JETHALAL

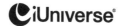

KUNDALINI YOGA MASSAGE
SEVEN STEPS TO ACTIVATE THE SEVEN CHAKRAS
AND POWER PEOPLE'S PRANA

Graphic credits to Daniel Yoshizawa of RG Digital Printing
1910 Kennedy RD. Unit # 3
Toronto, Ont M1P 2L8
Tel: (416) 292-4362
Fax: (416) 2920490
Email: rgdigital@gmail.com
Website: www.rgdigital.ca

iUniverse books may be ordered through booksellers or by contacting:

iUniverse
1663 Liberty Drive
Bloomington, IN 47403
www.iuniverse.com
1-800-Authors (1-800-288-4677)

ISBN: 978-1-4917-6607-1 (sc)
ISBN: 978-1-4917-6608-8 (hc)
ISBN: 978-1-4917-6609-5 (e)

Print information available on the last page.

iUniverse rev. date: 06/24/2015

Disclaimer

This book primarily focuses on integrating Kundalini yoga and massage to improve your overall health and well-being. *Kundalini yoga massage* should be performed by either a licensed registered massage therapist or someone trained in these techniques. The author and publisher are not responsible for any loss or suffering to the readers as a result of misuse of information provided herein.

"Hear now the Wisdom of Yoga,
The Yoga of Knowledge and Yoga of Action,
Path of the eternal and freedom from bondage.
No step is lost on the path and no dangers are found,
and even a little progress brings freedom from fear and
attainment of peace."

Bhagvad Gita

"The spirit dwelling in this body,
is really the same as the Supreme.
He has been spoken of as the Witness,
The Sustainer of all
The true Guide
The Experiencer,
The Overlord,
As well as the Absolute"

Bhagvad Gita

This book is dedicated to all known and unknown saints who gained enlightenment through their intense austerities and self-discipline. It is through their wisdom, knowledge and quest to find eternal universal truths thousands of years ago that we are able to become dedicated seekers of yoga today.

Although I have given credit to Leela Prasaud for her contribution in the acknowledgement section of the book, I would be failing in my duty if I did not inform the readers of her active participation from the inception of the book right through to its conclusion.

During the time of writing this book Leela's mum was critically ill and despite her own busy schedule Leela always rose up to the occasion to generously add her contributions. Leela's mum passed away on October 22, 2014 after blessing the first and original copy of the manuscript of *Kundalini Yoga Massage*.

Leela and I dedicate this book to both our mothers who, despite being widowed at a very early age, continued to be a shining light for their families. To our beloved mothers, our universal mother, and all mothers everywhere.

TABLE OF CONTENTS

FOREWORD

It is a privilege for me to write the foreword to Dr Gita Jethalal's book *Kundalini Yoga Massage* as I have personally experienced the incredible healing of this type of massage. Some of the techniques in *Kundalini Yoga Massge* have been around for thousands of years; however, after Western medicine gained prominence, these ancient techniques were only practised by a few people. The *Kundalini Yoga Massage* techniques are authentic. It is my hope that Gita's book will bring a revival of these techniques to complement other healing methods.

I have been blessed to be under the guidance of Swami Jyotirmayananda, a disciple of Swami Sivananda, for over twenty-five years. I have also been privileged to spend time at Swamiji's ashram in Miami. Swamiji is a living example of integral yoga which blends the four yogas of action, emotion, will and reason. Swamiji is one of the foremost proponents of integral yoga which results in personality integration. I practise Swamiji's teachings and was privileged to learn hatha yoga from Swamiji.

Practising yoga has made a tremendous difference in my life. I have seen the benefits in cancer patients who experience more energy through practising yoga and receiving treatments of *Kundalini Yoga Massage*. The elderly maintain better health and vitality through the practice of yoga. *Kundalini Yoga Massage* will further enhance their sense of well-being, as it taps into the powerful energy of the chakras.

Gita met Swamiji at our home shortly after she opened her chiropractic clinic. At that meeting Gita was delighted to receive Swamiji's blessing. I believe that the techniques of *Kundalini Yoga Massage* will further all healing processes by tapping into prana, the life force in all of us. The more people who have access to these techniques the greater will be the impact on health and well-being.

My prayers for everyone's good health, peace, and joy.

Leela Prasaud, yoga teacher

Divine blessings!

I am pleased to know that you have written the book, *Kundalini Yoga Massage*, focusing on removing physiological blockages from the areas around the seven chakras of Kundalini to assist patients and seekers of spiritual knowledge.

You are welcome to draw from my publications all that you need for your great project.

You have my permission to use my teachings for the benefit of all. You have my special blessings!

May God bless you with success!

With regards, Prem and Om,

Swami Jyotirmayananda
November 2014

PREFACE

I would like to take this opportunity to make the readers aware that traditionally activating or awakening one's Kundalini was seen to be a complex spiritual practice. Tradition dictated that aspirants who wished to awaken their Kundalini Shakti (power) required the guidance of a guru or spiritual master as a tremendous amount of discipline was required for the purification of the body and the mind as well as for strengthening the nervous system. The practice of raising one's Kundalini was confined to saints and sages; it was not meant to be practised by ordinary people and hence strict rules and regulations had to be adhered to.

However, I would also like to emphasise that "Kundalini" is the term used to describe the vital bioenergetic life force that lies dormant within all human beings until activated by the practice of yoga. From my own reading and experience I have come to understand that Kundalini is a primordial energy that exists in everyone; it is not necessary to isolate one's self from this material world to activate one's Kundalini. This dormant Kundalini power can be likened to the hidden generative power present in a seed. In order for the hidden power to be awakened within the seed it is necessary to plant the seed in healthy soil and create the ideal conditions required for the seed to grow and become a healthy plant. Unlike the seed, though, no apparent external physical changes are visible in humans. However, as a result of subtler changes that occur people become more balanced and integrated.

Unfortunately, many people are unaware of this creative, latent, potential energy and it continues to remain hidden. Throughout their lifetime people develop psychological and physiological blockages that prevent them from accessing this life force

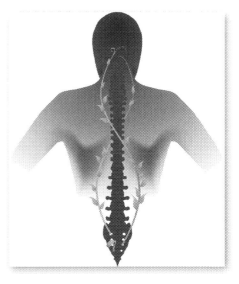

energy. A practitioner can access this dormant energy through the regular and disciplined practice of [1]yoga which includes the ancient techniques of postures (asanas), specialised, controlled breathing (pranayama), concentration and meditation. The massage techniques outlined in this book are designed to remove physiological blockages and also activate the life force energy that lies dormant at the base of the spine within all human beings.

There is a misconception among many people that the practice of yoga consists only of the asanas (postures). Thousands of years ago Sage Patanjali formulated an eight-step programme for living a balanced and ethical life. The asanas are only the third step of Patanjali's eight-step aphorisms. The postures improve flexibility and vitality by removing physiological blockages and prepare the body to remain seated in concentration and meditation for prolonged periods of time.

---

1   Whenever references are made to yoga throughout this book it is meant to include postures, controlled breathing techniques, concentration and meditation

In much the same way as the asanas remove physiological blockages, the techniques as outlined in seven-step *Kundalini Yoga Massage* become a first step to physiologically remove blockages from the chakras and activate the dormant bioenergetic life force. Combining *Kundalini Yoga Massage* and yoga and incorporating them into your lifestyle will create the ideal conditions and enable you to function as a unified whole. We are all aware that the journey of a thousand miles begins with a single step and mastering the techniques and practices outlined in *Kundalini Yoga Massage* is that very important first step on your journey to health, well-being and spiritual growth.

I am not saying that people can only awaken their dormant Kundalini (life force energy) by the techniques outlined in this book. They represent an important first step in one's life long journey. Internal self-evolution, self-discipline and determination are essential prerequisites to awakening one's Kundalini.

As mentioned earlier, this energy is inherently present within all of us and through self-discipline and the practice of yoga we all have equal opportunity of accessing this hidden energy and incorporating it into our daily lives. Of course, it is important to understand that like any investment that brings us high dividends, firm commitment and discipline are required.

I would also like to remove from the minds of the readers any misconception they may have associated with the term "Kundalini." In yogic tradition Kundalini describes the power of the divine having two aspects: one female, called Shakti, and the other, a male aspect referred to as Shiva. The female aspect is the dormant life force that is found at the base of the spine; once awakened, it can rise up to the crown of the head and unite with the male aspect, which is pure consciousness. This union is a symbolic representation of transcending limitations and dualities and expanding our individual consciousness to rise to its highest level and unite with the universal or cosmic consciousness bringing us to a state of ultimate bliss. This symbolism is sometimes misunderstood to represent sexual union. The ultimate premise of all forms of yoga is to unite our mind, body and soul; to transcend our senses and rise above limitations and dualities; and to expand our individual consciousness to unite with the universal consciousness.

For the purpose of this book, and for all intents and purposes, Kundalini is seen as the creative, intelligent, corporeal energy that exists within all human beings. I believe any misconception or sexual connotations come from misinterpretation or the lack of proper understanding. This book outlines steps that can be taken to unlock this dormant bioenergetic life force and the sole purpose of the book is to promote total well-being and the overall health benefits for millions of people.

REVIEW BY SWAMI JYOTIRMAYANANDA

By writing this excellent book, *Kundalini Yoga Massage (Seven-Steps to Activate the Seven Chakras and Power People's Prana)*, Dr Gita Jethalal has done an immense service to humanity. All the raging problems of the world are due to ill health, delusions of the intellect, distractions of the mind, agitations of pranas and absence of insight into spiritual values of life. In this book, the author has united the science of the West with the wisdom of the East; she offers a seven-step technique to perform Kundalini yoga massage along with all the needed insight to help everyone to enjoy health as the foundation of discovering all the spiritual potentiality of the soul. I extend my good wishes and blessings that by studying this book the readers may be inspired to practice the techniques, pursue the path of integral yoga, witness the blossoming of their soul and waft the fragrance of divine light, love and bliss!

May God shower His choicest blessings on Dr Gita Jethalal.

Sri Swami Jyotirmayananda

Swami Jyotirmayananda Personal Profile:

Swami Jyotirmayananda was initiated into the order of Sanyasa in 1953 by his guru, [1]Sri [2]Swami Sivananda, the founder of Divine Life Society in Rishikesh, India. Swamiji's great command of spiritual knowledge and dynamic expositions on yoga and Vedanta attracted enormous interest all over India.

In 1962, [3]Swamiji left India and travelled west to Puerto Rico to spread his wisdom and knowledge. Swamiji conducted regular classes in English and Spanish and made numerous television appearances while in Puerto Rico.

In March 1969, Swamiji moved to Miami and launched the Yoga Research Foundation and ashram. Today, there are several branches of this organisation worldwide.

In 1985, he established the International Yoga Society and the Divya Jyoti School in Loni near New Delhi. In 2000, the Jyotirmayananda Ashram and Vocational Training Centre for Abused and Neglected Women was established in Bihar, India. In 2006, the Lalita Jyoti Anathalaya, an orphanage and school, opened its doors for seventy-five girls in Sonipat. All the institutions in India serve the community through regular yoga classes, camps, children's schools and they operate free medical clinics.

Swami Jyotirmayananda is recognised as one of the foremost proponents of integral yoga. Swamiji continues to share his timeless wisdom via daily lectures in his Miami ashram as well as via live

---

1   Sri: is a term of respect for all males and also means revered.
2   Swami: is a title given to a Hindu Saint or a monk. In the eighth century
     Shankara reorganised India's ancient monastic order, and the members
     were called Swamis. A Swami is one who has taken a vow of celibacy and
     devoted himself to spiritual practices and serving humanity.
3   Swamiji: When the suffix ji is added to a name eg: Swamiji, it denotes
     added respect

podcasts online. He has authored numerous books and journals to help aspirants worldwide discover the secret wealth of self-realisation by tapping into the infinite power that is present within all human beings.

According to to Swami Paramahansa Yogananda, renowned author of *Autobiography of a Yogi*, "[1]Medicine, massage, spinal adjustments and electrical treatment bring back lost harmonious conditions to cells by physiological stimulation. These external methods assist to improve flow of prana and facilitate healing."

It is essential, however, to integrate in one's personal practice the external methods stated above with the internal disciplines of silence, concentration and meditation.

One of my favourite sayings from Desiderata is as follows:

> "Go placidly amidst the noise and the haste and remember what peace there may be in silence."

My personal equation for meditation, peace and rejuvenation is:

$$-\overline{n} + \overline{\xi} = \mathcal{E}^3$$

- N   (subtract or remove noise/external stimulation)
+ S   (add silence)
= E^3 (equates to accessing energy existing everywhere)

In his book *The Seven Spiritual Laws of Success*, renowned author and specialist in body-mind medicine, Dr. Deepak Chopra emphasises the need for silence and meditation. He says "[2]Through meditation you will learn to experience the field of pure silence and pure awareness."

1   Yogananda, Paramahansa, *Scientific Healings Affirmations*, 1981
2   Chopra, Deepak Dr., *The Seven Spiritual Laws of Success*, 1994

ACKNOWLEDGEMENTS

This book is a result of the collaborative effort of several dedicated people whose support and contributions led to its creation.

First and foremost I would like to thank Swami Jyotirmayananda for his blessings. Since a large part of this book is based on yoga philosophies I am grateful to Swamiji for giving me permission to use materials from his publications and for his guidance over the years. Swamiji is the founder of the Yoga Research Foundation in Miami and one of the foremost proponents of integral yoga. He is the living embodiment of spiritual wisdom of the Vedas which are ancient religious scriptures. Thank you, Swamiji, for your blessings. It means the world to me.

My gratitude goes out to Ms Cherry Aranzanso for her invaluable contribution in executing and perfecting the massage techniques outlined in this book.

My heartfelt thanks and gratitude go out to Ms Lina Totino for putting up with my illegible handwriting and trying to decipher what I meant to say in legible typewritten script. Without Lina's patience, persistence and tenacity this book would not have become a reality. Thank you so much, Lina. Thanks also to Wendy Chen and Dr Peter Kwong and Susan Loi for their contributions.

I am grateful to Leela Prasaud who reviewed the yoga sections of this book. Leela is one of Swami Jyotirmayananda's long-time devotees who has been leading hatha yoga, meditation and study groups in the greater Toronto area for over twenty years. I have known Leela for the past two decades and she always generously shares her wisdom, love and divinity whenever we meet. Thank you and bless you, Leela.

I also wish to thank Daniel Yoshizawa, Jay, and the staff at RG Digital for designing the cover and the layout of the book. It was Daniel's expertise and creativity that transformed the book and breathed life into it. We are all deeply indebted to you, Daniel, and thanks again.

My heartfelt thanks go to the very competent staff at iUniverse for their skilful editing. It was a pleasure dealing with the staff at all levels. I would wholeheartedly recommend iUniverse to any potential author.

My sincere thanks go to Danika Sherman for her suggestions.

Last but not least I wish to thank my husband, Madhukar, and son, Prashant, for their patience, understanding and support and for allowing me to pursue my dreams and to live life on my own terms.

I also wish to thank my husband for reviewing the book and for all his useful suggestions and recommendations. I sincerely appreciate your time and effort.

I love you all and am truly blessed to be surrounded by kind and considerate people.

INTRODUCTION

Living in the modern world with technological advancements that we could not even have dreamt of twenty to thirty years ago gives us unprecedented opportunities and resources to shape our world. Modern technology is keeping humanity globally interconnected but this also means that our obsession and dependence on technology has made it mandatory for many people to be available 24/7, to respond to emails and texts and to keep up with the numerous social media sites that are now available.

Technological advancements have their place; they have made life infinitely more convenient and brought distant people and places closer than ever. They have revolutionised health care, changed politics and affected our lives in every way imaginable. But, technological advancements have also increased alienation and led many to become obsessed with the latest gadgets. This obsession becomes time consuming and leads us to neglect other areas of our lives and consequently our health and well-being are compromised.

Many of us spend more time servicing our cars and appliances than we do paying attention to our health and well-being. The cumulative effect of the numerous stressors in our daily lives takes its toll on our bodies and leaves us worn out and prone to dysfunction and disease.

If we wish to continue to be productive and maintain our health it is imperative that we find the time to take preventative measures to remain fit and functional in all areas of our lives. If we don't pay attention to our physical and mental needs and reduce our stressors in a timely way then I am afraid that humans and technology are heading towards a collision course.

I found that combining the regular, disciplined practice of yoga with therapeutic massage is a very useful form of preventative maintenance. Just like everyone else, I too was caught in the web of trying to be productive and perfect in multiple areas of my life. I soon realised that trying to change the different parameters of my external life was too demanding because new challenges kept cropping up every day.

Over the years, I have tried several different self-help techniques and tools to strengthen my inner self; each technique was a stepping stone in my spiritual journey. Without a shadow of a doubt, the greatest success in my journey of self-discovery came when I made the practice of yoga and meditation an integral part of my lifestyle. I continued living the same busy life but as I changed from within my external circumstances and surroundings changed simultaneously.

I am now putting out less effort and accomplishing a lot more in a peaceful and purposeful manner. I wholeheartedly attribute the positive changes that occurred in my life to the "magic" of yoga. I have experienced first-hand the benefits of yoga and massage and after being in the health care field for over forty years I decided to write this book on *Kundalini Yoga Massage.*

Many people believe that to experience the power of Kundalini yoga they should study under a trained teacher. I agree that for aspirants who wish to fast-track their spiritual evolution a trained teacher is necessary. However, the techniques in this book are essentially intended for people who wish to take charge of their health, well-being, peace and spiritual growth. It must be noted that personal health, overall well-being and major life goals require an on-going effort. This book must be viewed as only the first step in a lifelong effort. It is essential that one takes charge of one's health and well-being and not be dependant solely on the help of gurus or spiritual masters. Outside help and guidance will prove ineffective if one does not implement what is shared and taught by others. There is no substitute for on-going personal effort which often times requires fundamental life style changes.

Kundalini Yoga Massage combines the wisdom and philosophy of yoga with the therapeutic benefits of massage therapy. The Seven-step Kundalini yoga massage focuses on stimulating the paraspinal soft tissue areas around the individual chakras which are subtle energy centres within the spinal column. According to yogic philosophy, Kundalini refers to the corporeal or potential energy that lies dormant at the base of the spine until activated by the practice of yoga. *Kundalini Yoga Massage* assists in removing physiological blockages and increasing the flow of life force energy (prana). Swami Paramahansa Yogananda, renowned author of *Autobiography of a Yogi*, so rightly said, "Medicine, massage, spinal adjustments and electrical treatment bring back lost harmonious conditions to cells by physiological stimulation. These external methods assist to improve the flow of prana and facilitate healing."

Yoga asanas (postures) focus on the gross movements of the spine to stimulate the flow of life force energy whilst Kundalini yoga massage increases the flow of pranic energy at a much subtler level by direct physiological intervention. Changes at a subtler level are more enduring and effective.

The principles of this book are based on yoga, ancient yogic philosophy and massage therapy. Since yoga deals with the overall health of a person as a unified whole it surpasses all other forms of self-improvement techniques that are currently available. Although the book presents a seven-step technique to activate the seven chakras it is not necessary to be a registered massage therapist to incorporate these techniques into your lifestyle, unless, of course, you wish to use it professionally. For people who wish to use seven-step Kundalini yoga massage for personal use I suggest taking a weekend workshop to familiarise yourself with the basics.

If you have tried practising yoga asanas and having a regular massage, I urge you to incorporate *Kundalini Yoga Massage* into your routine. It integrates several new and innovative techniques to improve your energy levels and take your health and your yoga practice to an elevated level. The techniques as outlined in this book will improve your life on multiple levels and instead of being constantly stressed out you will begin to live and enjoy the life that you always imagined. It is my hope that *Kundalini Yoga Massage* will become a lifetime regime for millions of people ensuring good health, increasing well-being and enhancing their ability to deal with stress.

CHAPTER 1:
WHY ANOTHER BOOK ON YOGA?

In the past few decades, the practice of yoga has become popular and widespread, especially in the West. There are hundreds, if not thousands, of different styles and adaptations of yoga today. However, irrespective of the different styles of yoga they all share one underlying quality in that they provide many benefits to the individuals who practise it.

Whether you are a beginner or a master, yoga practitioners are able to experience palpable benefits. These benefits give millions of people an incentive to make the practice of yoga an integral part of their lifestyle. Why is it that yoga has such a beneficial effect on human beings? Yoga is a system of self-development that encourages the body, mind and spirit to act as one unit and become harmoniously integrated. Through yoga we develop a heightened awareness that our physical actions affect our mental outlook and vice versa. Yoga also helps us to unlock the life force energy that lies hidden within us and opens up the secret doorway to self-discovery and self-realisation.

Yoga today has become a multimillion-dollar business and the stores are overflowing with books, CDs, DVDs, clothing and accessories to improve and enhance one's yoga practice.

Books on yoga are abundantly available, so why another book on yoga? There are many reasons why this book is different: The first reason is that *Kundalini Yoga Massage* focuses on a new and innovative way of activating the seven chakras to unlock the flow of the inherent, latent energy found within human beings. It also integrates two ancient arts, yoga and massage, to improve our overall health and well-being. There are several books written on the different aspects of yoga. Most of these books focus on the physical aspects of yoga and on the specialised breathing techniques both of which are an integral part of yoga practice. Since the recent rise in the popularity of yoga a number of books have been written on the different types and adaptations of yoga and their historical significance.

Despite the wide range of books that are available on yoga there are very few books that actually focus on the science behind why yoga works. This book is different from those other books because it focuses on human anatomy and physiology, particularly on the neuromuscular system, and explains the science behind why yoga works from both Western and Eastern points of view. If we have a basic understanding of how our human body works and an understanding of yogic philosophy and how it can be integrated into our daily lives then we will more readily incorporate it into our everyday routine.

This, then, becomes one of the most important areas in which this book differs from other books on yoga. *Kundalini Yoga Massage* applies various combinations of different techniques that follow the basic principles of yogic philosophy and massage therapy. Thai yoga massage and traditional ancient Ayurvedic massage are excellent massage therapy techniques that are also based on yoga and yogic philosophy. However, Kundalini Yoga Massage, whose techniques are also based on yogic philosophy, is unique because the techniques activate the seven chakras by direct physiological intervention. The basic premise of yoga is to activate this bioenergetic, intelligent life force that is latent in all human beings and *Kundalini Yoga Massage* directly incorporates this premise making it a very effective modality to include in your quest for good health.

Many people have attempted to understand the wisdom of ancient philosophies and found them too abstract. I agree that some ancient concepts are difficult to grasp and our good intention to apply these philosophies falls by the wayside. This has been my own personal experience and I know that I am not alone. The ancient yogic philosophies were formulated over five thousand years ago and are sometimes difficult for present-day readers to understand and assimilate. My aim in writing this book was to simplify some of the abstract philosophies so it is easier for readers to incorporate them into their lifestyle.

Many of us have difficulty in believing that we function in a disjointed way with our body, mind and soul being pulled in different directions. Unbeknown to many, there lies at the base of the spine of all human beings a vital, bioenergetic force that is similar to the potential energy contained within a seed, waiting to be accessed so that it can unfold and blossom. It is through the practice of yoga that this inherent life force energy can be activated and incorporated as an asset in our daily lives.

Furthermore, in recent times, there has been an interest in combining the knowledge of Western science with the ancient wisdom of the East and throughout the book this East/West unity is emphasised. The state-of-the-art technology developed in the West gives us access to enormous amounts of educational information at the touch of a button and this technology can become an important tool for learning new techniques to improve our lives.

As yoga becomes more and more mainstream, numerous studies are being conducted to gauge its efficacy in treating a host of medical ailments. Yoga has a beneficial effect on multiple levels and has been shown to increase our overall flexibility and strength, boost the immune system and decrease stress.

The techniques outlined in this book will not only provide a novel method to increase the flow of your life force energy (prana), but will also assist you in dealing with the stressors of modern society more efficiently and improve all areas of your life.

This book differs from other yoga books because it makes a concerted effort to unify the wisdom of the East with the science and technology of the West for the benefit of mankind. This book is also unique because it not only embodies the theory and the science behind why yoga works it also provides a practical, seven-step technique to incorporate *Kundalini Yoga Massage* into your lifestyle as a foundation to build better health.

CHAPTER 2:
OUR AMAZING NERVOUS SYSTEM
AND HOW IT FUNCTIONS

In order to understand the benefits of yoga and *Kundalini Yoga Massage* and how it can positively impact your health and wellbeing it is necessary to have a basic understanding of the nervous system and the muscular system and how they relate to yoga. Of course, the body has several other systems which work closely together to keep our body healthy and functional. However, for the purpose of this book we are focusing on the nervous system and muscular system and how they are intricately aligned for us to perform even the simplest action.

The fundamentals and foundations of yogic philosophy are based on the premise that a well-maintained and balanced nervous system is the core of a fully integrated human being. This book focuses on the practice of Kundalini yoga as it is directly linked to the nervous system. Kundalini is the innate intelligent energy that exists within all of us and lies dormant at the base of the spine until activated by the practice of yoga which includes postures (asanas), specialised breathing (pranayama) and meditation. This in-dwelling energy can now also be activated physiologically by the techniques outlined in this book. In order to fully appreciate the efficacy of yoga and its role in our health and well-being it is important to understand how stress and stressors directly affect the nervous system and how this consequently becomes the underlying cause of a variety of diseases in the body.

The nervous system is the most important system in the body since it tells the rest of the body what to do and how to work together in a co-ordinated manner. The nervous system is a highly complex, integrated system but for the purpose of this book we will simplify both form and function in an easy-to-understand manner. A complex network of billions of microscopic cells called neurons make up the nervous system. The neurons connect with each other to form neural pathways that bundle up together to carry messages back and forth via electrochemical impulses, like wires in a telephone exchange.

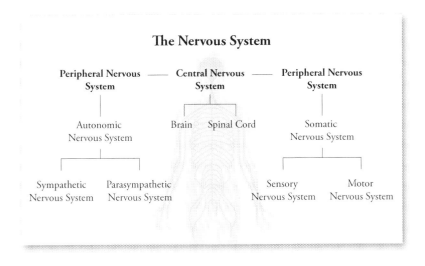

The Nervous System

Peripheral Nervous System	Central Nervous System	Peripheral Nervous System
Autonomic Nervous System	Brain Spinal Cord	Somatic Nervous System
Sympathetic Nervous System Parasympathetic Nervous System		Sensory Nervous System Motor Nervous System

The nervous system is made up of the central nervous system and the peripheral nervous system. The central nervous system is made up of the brain and spinal cord and is housed within the cavities of the cranium and spinal column, respectively. The peripheral nervous system lies outside of the cranium and spinal column. The main function of the peripheral nervous system is to connect the central nervous system to the limbs and organs. The peripheral nervous system is further subdivided into the somatic nervous system and the autonomic nervous system. The somatic nervous system is responsible for receiving external stimuli as well as co-ordinating body movements.

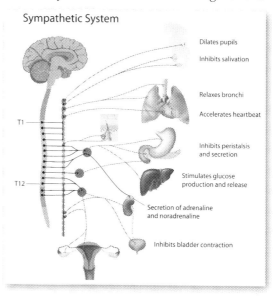

Sympathetic System

Dilates pupils

Inhibits salivation

Relaxes bronchi

Accelerates heartbeat

Inhibits peristalsis and secretion

Stimulates glucose production and release

Secretion of adrenaline and noradrenaline

Inhibits bladder contraction

It is the system that regulates activities that are under our conscious control. The autonomic nervous system is further subdivided into the sympathetic nervous system and the parasympathetic system.

The sympathetic nervous system, which operates below the conscious level, is designed to be activated as a defence mechanism during times of impending danger. This system is responsible for increasing blood pressure, respiration rate, heart rate and other physiological changes that are activated during the fight-or-flight response. When the fight-or-flight response is activated the blood flow is diverted from non-essential parts of the body to essential parts where they are needed.

Unfortunately, the stressors of everyday living in the fast-paced modern society have caused our bodies to be in a habitual state of fight-or-flight mode. Panic, anxiety, fear and all other daily stressors cause an increase in levels of stress hormones such as adrenaline and cortisol which are activated during the fight-or-flight response and this has a negative effect on our nervous system.

The autonomic nervous system is normally considered not to be under our conscious control. According to yogic philosophy by practising the asanas, pranayama and meditative techniques you can consciously gain control of your breath and slow down your breathing and your heart rate. In yoga the breath is likened to a switch that controls the engine, which is the body. By consciously controlling the switch we can gain control of our body and we can subsequently not only achieve excellent physical health but improve our mental capacity as well.

The parasympathetic nervous system, on the other hand, has the

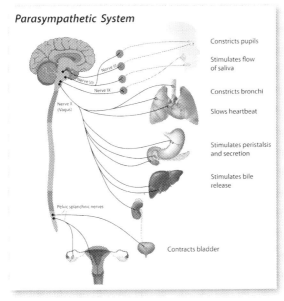

Parasympathetic System

Constricts pupils

Stimulates flow of saliva

Nerve III

Nerve VII

Nerve IX

Constricts bronchi

Nerve X (Vagus)

Slows heartbeat

Stimulates peristalsis and secretion

Stimulates bile release

Pelvic splanchnic nerves

Contracts bladder

opposite effect of the sympathetic nervous system. Activating the parasympathetic nervous system slows down the heart rate, lowers the blood pressure, decreases the respiration rate and returns the body's function to normal rest-and-repair mode.

When practising any aspect of yoga, be it the asanas, pranayama or any meditative technique we are consciously activating the parasympathetic nervous system and switching our bodies to the rest-and-repair mode, a state that brings us optimal health. By bringing our breath under our conscious control we start a series of physiological events that activates the parasympathetic nervous system. Dr Herbert Benson, founder of Mind-Body Medical

Institute of Harvard University, has done extensive clinical studies with Buddhist monks to confirm what he calls the "relaxation response."[1]

Most of us are unaware that the nervous system is a very specialised system that acts as a photographic plate in which our daily experiences (via our thoughts and actions) are recorded in much the same way as a photograph is developed. According to yogic philosophy the thoughts and actions recorded on the nervous system become impressions on our neural pathway. These impressions are called samskaras.

Through improved diagnostic imaging we can now view the internal architecture and function of the brain in greater detail and with greater accuracy. Modern technology and diagnostic imaging have enabled scientists and researchers to make enormous strides in understanding the mechanism behind neuroplasticity[2] which refers to the ability of the brain and spinal cord to reorganise itself. Research shows scientific evidence that the brain has the ability to form new neural connections through axonal sprouting, neurogenesis, and this can occur throughout adult life. Neurogenesis is the process by which new nerve cells are generated. Neuroplasticity allows nerve cells to compensate for injury or disease and readjust their activities in response to changes in the environment.

Modern research now validates yogic philosophy which states that through the practice of yoga, focusing on asanas, controlled breathing and meditation we can access subtle life force energies (prana) that can help us to form new neural pathways and help us literally remodel our brain. Meditation helps us erase worn out thoughts and misbeliefs and create new thoughts, memories and

1   Dr Herbert Benson, *The Relaxation Response.*
2   Dr. Norman Doidge, *The Brain that Changes Itself.*

beliefs that will be beneficial for our health and well-being.[3] Dr. Andrew Newburg a neuroscientist and a pioneer in neurological study of religious and spiritual practices, scanned the brains of Tibetian Buddhist meditators, and discovered that there was a decreased activity in the area of the parietal lobe during meditation. As a result of the experiment he arrived at the hypothesis "that blocking all sensory and cognitive input in this area during meditation is associated with a sense of no space and no time that is so often is described in meditation." We come to the realisation that the combined practice of yoga, including meditation, can literally allow us to rewrite the script of our lives.

Kundalini yoga is a meditative discipline that gives special consideration to the spine and nervous system thus creating a direct communication between the mind and body to facilitate healing. Since Kundalini is the primordial life force energy within the body it is the source of physical, emotional and spiritual healing when activated.

Whether we look at how the nervous system works from the viewpoint of Western science or from the perspective of Eastern philosophy's primordial core energy, it is predominately clear that the negative effects of stress cause dysfunction in the nervous system. Since the nervous system acts like a giant telephone exchange and innervates the entire body a dysfunction in the nervous system has far-reaching effects in other parts of the physical body as well as the mind.

In this day and age with our very busy lifestyles what tools do we have to deal with our daily stressors? Unfortunately, we do not have a magic pill that can relieve our stress. The only non-invasive viable option to deal with stress is through the practice of yoga which, as

3   Dr Andrew Newberg, *Andrewnewburg.com.* *"How do meditation and prayer change our brain?"*

stated earlier, includes exercise or physical postures, specialised breathing techniques, concentration and meditation.

The techniques as outlined in this book are based on yogic philosophy and are designed to activate the seven chakras by physiological means and together with the practice of yoga they become a very important modality to reduce stress and promote a healthy body and mind. This is achieved by activating the bioenergetic energy that lies latent in all human beings.

The techniques outlined in this book not only dissipate the negative effects of stress on the nervous system but also encourages mind-body integration. The efficacy of mind-body medicine is well researched and mind-body programmes are well established at several prestigious universities all over the world.

CHAPTER 3:
OUR VERSATILE MUSCULAR
SYSTEM AND A BRIEF DESCRIPTION
OF HOW IT FUNCTIONS

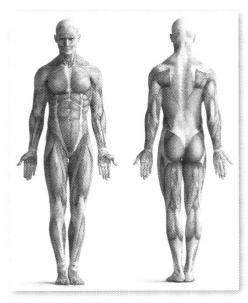

The muscular system is responsible for movement in the human body. Muscles are attached to the skeletal system; people have over seven hundred muscles which make up roughly half the total body weight.

There are three major types of muscles, namely visceral, cardiac and skeletal muscles. The visceral and cardiac muscles which make up our heart and other organs are known as involuntary muscles as they are not directly controlled by the conscious mind.

On the other hand, the skeletal muscles which are under our conscious control work together with the bones and joints to form a lever system whose main function is movement. Muscle tone keeps the muscles partially contracted and is responsible for maintaining and upholding the body's posture throughout the day, without fatigue.

Nerve cells bundled together called motor neurons control several muscle cells. Together, they are called a motor unit. When a motor neuron receives a signal from the brain it stimulates all the muscle cells in its motor unit at the same time. Nerve impulses cause a motor unit to contract. Muscles always contract before relaxing. Not all muscle contractions produce movement. In an isotonic contraction the tension remains unchanged whilst only the muscle length shortens and lengthens. The shortening phase is called "concentric" whereas the lengthening phase is called "eccentric". A bicep curl using a weight is an example of isotonic contraction. Bending the elbow is a concentric contraction and extending the elbow is an eccentric contraction.

When people tense their bodies due to stress, anger or fear they are performing an isometric contraction. An isometric contraction is a static contraction without any visible movement in the joint meaning that the length of the muscle and the angle of the joint do not change. For moderate levels of force muscles use aerobic respiration which requires oxygen to fuel cellular activities and is more efficient. For higher levels of force the muscles use anaerobic respiration where no oxygen is required; this method is less efficient and causes muscles to tire more easily.

The human body is designed anatomically and physiologically to react to stress and the reaction of the body to stress can affect the person physically, emotionally and mentally. When a person is unable to manage the stress and there is an accumulated build-up of stress without relief then distress or disease sets in.

When we are stressed out our bodies, especially our muscles, tense up and prepare us for a fight-or-flight response. Continual stress causes muscles and other parts of the body to be in a state of chronic fight-or-flight mode and this leads to muscle fatigue and exhaustion. Massage therapy assists in releasing and relaxing tight muscles to improve circulation and speed up healing. Remember that muscles make up over half our body weight so keeping our muscular system relaxed, healthy and tension free is a prerequisite for health and well-being. The yoga postures and the techniques discussed in this book play an important role in keeping the muscular system tension free. The slow, rhythmical stretches of the asanas require the use of muscles and this stretching is the key to relaxing and releasing energy and improving flexibility. These asanas are performed with great awareness and deep concentration and each posture is designed to unlock the hidden life force energy and physically prepare the body for concentration and meditation.

Kundalini Yoga Massage incorporates several manual massage techniques to remove physiological blockages from the energy centres (chakras) and energy channels (nadis) and encourages the dormant vibratory energy that lies latent at the base of the spine to be activated. Activation of the chakras revitalises the physical body, relaxes the muscles and accelerates body-mind-soul integration.

CHAPTER 4:
DYSFUNCTION OF THE NEUROMUSCULAR SYSTEM AND HOW IT AFFECTS US

In the preceding chapter we briefly outlined the nervous and muscular systems and described how these systems are intricately aligned to perform even the simplest action.

The muscular and nervous systems assist each other to perform their respective motor and sensory functions. Muscles not only protect the delicate network of nerves that innervate the body they also provide the brain with valuable information about controlling the body's movements via electrochemical impulses. The nervous system transmits nerve impulses which are responsible for every movement and function in our body and this even includes our thoughts. Neither skeletal muscles nor smooth or cardiac muscles would be able to function if their connections to the nerves were disrupted or severed. It is these thread-like nerves that bring power to the muscles.

In an ideal stress-free world all the systems in a healthy individual should be working optimally. Unfortunately, injury, trauma, stress and poor posture all cause dysfunction in the transmission of the nerve impulses resulting in the body going into a state disequilibrium or disease. Massage therapy has been used to partially address this disequilibrium by mobilising the body's soft tissue. Soft tissue incorporates muscles, tendons and connective tissue. Kundalini yoga massage therapy helps to bring back balance to the nervous system by rehabilitating the soft tissue, activating the seven chakras by unleashing the dormant energy that lies latent at the base of the spine and this improves our overall health and function.

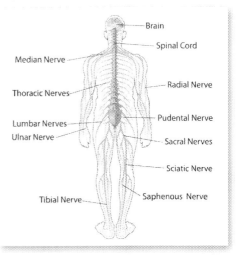

The adverse effect of stress, trauma, injury and poor posture can result in neuromuscular dysfunctions. In order to assess the extent of muscular dysfunction it is important to do an initial biomechanical gait analysis to isolate any postural distortions and nerve entrapments with the goal of

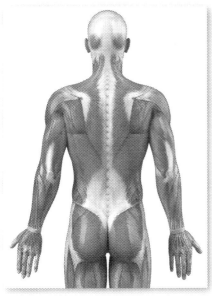

preventing any further postural damage. All skeletal muscles work in opposite pairs meaning that whilst one muscle contracts the other relaxes. These muscles are referred to as "agonist and antagonist." The opposing nature in which the muscles work causes undue tension and stress in multiple areas. This in turn causes postural dysfunction; the connective tissues get restricted, impeding both spinal movements and the flow of life force energy (prana).

Dysfunction impedes the proper flow of life force energy and puts the body into a state of disease. Yoga asanas and Kundalini yoga massage are designed to help relieve the tension in the neuromuscular system and help us relax both physically and mentally.

CHAPTER 5:
BASIC DIFFERENCE BETWEEN WESTERN MASSAGE THERAPY AND EASTERN MASSAGE THERAPY

There are several different types of massages using a variety of techniques and modalities. Massage therapy has been used by different cultures all over the world for therapeutic benefits. The origin of massage therapy dates back thousands of years.

Today, different massage techniques are used to treat a variety of health-related problems. The spectrum of reasons for having a massage may range from pure relaxation to reducing stress and tension to treating more complex problems such as tension headaches and injury rehabilitation.

In Western society one of the most common forms of massage therapy is Swedish massage. Swedish massage combines a variety of massage techniques to break down adhesions or restrictions within muscles and connective tissues. Swedish massage is the foundation for a number of different types of massages including aromatherapy, relaxation massage, full body massage and sports massage. Swedish massage can be either gentle or a more vigorous type of deep tissue massage. The therapist may decide to use a combination of gentle and vigorous massage techniques depending on the patient's need. The intensity of the massage depends on the patient's requirements and pain tolerance. All the techniques in Swedish massage focus on releasing chronic muscle tension by breaking down adhesions in muscles and connective tissues.

The different types of massage in the Western world are based on the gross anatomy and physiology of the human body and they are not based on activating the subtle energy centres which is the essence of Eastern styles of massage. According to Eastern philosophies chi and prana are life force energies that exist within the body. These life force energies flow in subtle, invisible meridians or channels. A dysfunction or disruption of the flow of energy manifests as a dysfunction in the body's organs.

The Chinese philosophy focuses on meridians which are passages through which the chi and blood circulate. On the other hand, the Indian philosophy, which is based on yogic philosophy, focuses on the nadis and chakras which are subtle, invisible energy channels and energy centres through which vital life force energy flows. It must be emphasised that both the traditional Chinese massage techniques and the Indian massage techniques will improve the flow of life force energy and will provide many benefits for a patient's overall well-being. However, since this book focuses on *Kundalini Yoga Massage* we will be focusing on yogic philosophy and its overall benefits.

Thai yoga massage and Ayurvedic massage are also based on yogic philosophy. However, unlike other massage techniques, *Kundalini Yoga Massage* focuses on a direct physiological intervention of removing blockages from the energy centres and energy channels thereby activating the flow of vital life force energy. During the practice of different yoga postures, techniques and meditation the very same vital life force energy is activated. The palpable benefit of increasing the flow of vital energy is the very reason why millions of people all over the world have made yoga an integral part of their lifestyle. In order to fully grasp the beneficial effects of yoga and yoga massage it is important to have a basic understanding of how stress affects the neuromuscular system. The cumulative effect of the stressors in our daily lives, be they work related, personal or otherwise, has an adverse impact on our neuromuscular system, causing our muscles to tense up and dulling our minds.

There is widespread awareness of the pivotal role that yoga plays in uniting our body mind and soul and allowing us to function in a more integrated way. The techniques outlined in *Kundalini Yoga Massage* form the foundation of a very important modality that assists the body and mind to relax and thereby decrease tension. Chapter 10 gives a more detailed analysis of how stress affects the nervous system.

In the earlier chapters we gave a brief and basic description of the nervous system and muscular system, how they function and their role in Kundalini yoga massage. It must be remembered that with *Kundalini Yoga Massage* you not only enjoy all the benefits of traditional massage but you also have the added benefit of improving the flow of vital life force energy by activating the seven chakras.

CHAPTER 6:
THE BENEFITS OF MASSAGE THERAPY AND KUNDALINI YOGA MASSAGE

Massage therapy is a comprehensive intervention involving a range of techniques to mobilise soft tissue and joints of the body. According to [1]Canada's Massage Therapy Act of 1991, the purpose of massage therapy is to "prevent, develop, maintain, rehabilitate or augment physical function or relieve pain." Massage therapy is a clinically oriented health option that assists in pain relief from a variety of stressors including muscular overuse and chronic pain syndrome. A practitioner of massage therapy is called a registered licensed massage therapist.

Prior to a massage session a patient's full history is initially obtained and diagnostic tests reviewed. During the massage a therapeutic relationship is established between the patient and the practitioner who both work towards a common and realistic goal. Whether your goal is to enjoy a moment of relaxation, reduce muscle tension, obtain relief from chronic pain or improve joint function a therapeutic massage has been shown to provide a wide variety of benefits.

As the numerous health benefits of massage therapy have become widely accepted, the use of massage therapy has grown rapidly in recent times. The benefits of massage therapy are too

---

1   Massage Therapy Act 1991, SO 1991, c 27 s 3

numerous for us to discuss in detail. For the purposes of this book we will enumerate only the major benefits.

1. Improves flexibility and range of motion in joints
2. Relaxes muscles and relieves stress
3. Improves posture as major postural muscles are relaxed during massage
4. Improves circulation and lowers blood pressure
5. Removes toxins and encourages lymphatic drainage
6. Relieves tension headaches
7. Accelerates recovery after an injury or surgery
8. Strengthens the immune system

With Kundalini yoga massage you will enjoy all the numerous benefits of regular massage. In addition, Kundalini yoga massage releases nerve entrapments, improves breathing and stimulates the energy centres (chakras) and activates them which then improves the flow of life force energy (prana). Kundalini yoga massage activates the peripheral nervous system which slows down the heart rate, lowers the blood pressure and slows down the breathing rate. This leads to deep physical and mental relaxation.

Both Kundalini yoga massage and hatha yoga asanas will assist in removing physiological blockages from the areas surrounding the chakras and the nadis. However, Kundalini yoga massage has an added advantage of a more direct physiological intervention as it addresses each of the seven chakras individually. As mentioned earlier, Kundalini energy is primordial energy that lies dormant until activated by the practice of yoga, hatha yoga or stimulated by Kundalini yoga massage. This improves the flow of prana, helps increase energy levels and enhances vitality. It will improve not only your overall yoga practice but also your health and well-being by uniting your body, mind and soul to function as a fully integrated being.

CHAPTER 7:
A BRIEF DISCUSSION ON THE DIFFERENT TYPES OF YOGA

In Sanskrit *yoga* means "yoke" or union of the body, mind and soul. Yoga, therefore, is an integrated system of self-development involving mental and physical training. It is through the disciplined and ancient practice of yoga that the saints and sages of great intellectual stature came to understand that human beings in general do not function as integrated, unified beings. Judging from our external appearance we all appear whole but on closer examination we find that our body, mind, heart, soul and emotions seem to be pulling us in different directions. Our modern lifestyle seems to have exacerbated this disjointed phenomenon as we are always trying to play catch-up to keep our external world in order and subsequently neglecting our inner being.

The wise old yogis understood that this diversity of function in human beings could have an adverse effect on their personality and subsequently affect their lives negatively. In order to counteract this disjointedness the yogis formulated yoga to integrate people's body, mind and soul. The ancient art of yoga was practised and perfected in India thousands of years ago. The practice of yoga emphasises right living and the teachings were based on universal truths that are as valid today as they were thousands of years ago.

In the ancient Hindu scriptures there is a description of several types of yoga but for the purposes of this book we will focus on the five main paths. Four of these paths correspond to the four aspects of human personality: action, emotion, will and reason. When the four aspects of the human personality are practised as integral yoga, the personality becomes integrated. Aspirants can choose any combination of the paths of yoga that is suited to their personality and through sincere practice they will discover not only their true nature but also the extraordinary powers of their untapped potential.

Listed below are the five main branches of yoga that have evolved over the centuries:

1. **Karma yoga** (the yoga of action) is the path of correct action. This path converts karma (action) to karma yoga by the attitude of performing selfless action for the good of all. During this process thought patterns are changed. When a person's thought patterns change the mind becomes purified and the person becomes peaceful.

2. **Bhakti yoga** (the yoga of devotion) allows the feelings to be uplifted which brings about emotional integration in the person. Unlike other practices that require specific qualifications bhakti yoga is natural to everyone as we all know love. Through the practice of bhakti yoga, you gain insight into the nature of emotions and sentiment including how to deal with emotions in a mature way.

3. **Raja yoga** (the yoga of meditation) is the profound study of the mind which gives you deep insight into psychology of human nature. Sage Patanjali compiled eight steps leading to right living and a balanced mind. The eight steps are the virtues of good conduct, observances, and austerities; practice of physical postures and controlled breathing; withdrawal of the senses; concentration; meditation; and

Samadhi (super consciousness). Through the practice of Raja yoga you learn to control the body, mind and senses and you change negative thought patterns by directing the will to a more positive way of viewing situations. This allows you to develop a strong will and a controlled mind. Throughout the book frequent reference is made to the physical postures (asanas), specialised breathing techniques (pranayama), concentration and meditation. The brief synopsis of the four steps that follows will give the reader a better understanding of four aphorisms as outlined by Sage Patanjali's eight-fold path of the yoga sutras. For the purpose of the book we only focus on four of the eight steps of Patanjali's yoga sutras. For readers who wish to understand all eight steps I recommend *Sacred Wisdom: The Yoga Sutras of Patanjali*, translation and introduction by Swami Vivekananda. Listed below are four of the eight steps of Patanjali's yoga sutras:

Third Step of the Yoga Sutras
Physical Postures (Asanas): Different postures promote the flow of life force energy within the spinal column and this energy is then distributed to other parts of the body via the chakras (energy centres) and nadis (energy channels). Asanas are important to keep the body flexible, healthy and tension free. The regular practice of asanas strengthens the body and allows one to remain seated in a meditative pose for a prolonged period of time. Many beginners mistakenly think that the practice of yoga asanas constitutes the entire practice of yoga. However, this is not the case as yoga asanas are only the third step in Patanjali's eight-fold path of the yoga sutras.

Fourth Step of the Yoga Sutras

Specialised Breathing Techniques: Pranayama is the fourth step in the eight-fold path of the yoga sutras. Pranayama is the science of controlled breathing which accounts for the reception and distribution of cosmic life force energy. Through specialised breathing exercises which focus on proper inhalation and exhalation aspirants are able to gain control of their thoughts and subsequently their mind. Regular practice of mastering breath control results in an increased reception of life force energy and through prolonged exhalation during pranayama aspirants are able to get rid of stale, deoxygenated air. This assists in cleansing and purifying the blood and nervous system which subsequently leads to having a healthy body, mind and soul.

Sixth and Seventh Steps of the Yoga Sutras

Concentration and Meditation: Meditation is the culmination of the process of inner reflection. A dull and distracted mind does not possess clarity of thought or reason. Prior to reaching a state of deep meditation it is necessary to practice concentration, or one pointedness, where the mind is trained to concentrate on one point or idea. The practice of concentration is similar to focusing the rays of the sun via a lens onto a sheet of paper.[1] When the rays of the sun are scattered it is barely possible to even warm the paper but when the rays are focused on one point via the lens we can actually ignite the paper. A similar effect is possible during concentration when

---

1   Swami Jyotirmayananda, *Concentration and Meditation* (International Yoga Society, 2013).

the mind is focused on one thought, object or idea and nothing else occupies the entire field of consciousness.

Meditation: Meditation is the state of consciousness where the meditator is in a state of "thoughtless awareness"; this state can only be understood at a direct, intuitive level. Our ordinary, everyday experiences are limited by time, space and causal laws, whereas in a meditative state we transcend all boundaries. Meditation is a state where one experiences profound peace and the mind is silent, still and in a state of complete bliss and yet alert. Meditation is a continuous flow of one's perception, uninterrupted, along one channel; it can be likened to continuously pouring oil from one vessel into another. There are many different types of meditative techniques but for the purpose of this book we will focus on Kundalini meditation.

During Kundalini meditation the aspirant focuses on each chakra and also on uncoiling of the latent primordial energy that lies dormant at the base of the spine.[2] According to Swami Jyotirmayananda, meditation is absolutely essential to cross the vast realm of the unconscious mind and attain heights of sublime peace, bliss and self-realisation.

4. **Kundalini yoga**: *"Kundalini"* is a Sanskrit word that means "coiled." The word *"Kunda"* also means a bowl in which we ignite fire and this fire becomes the symbolic unleashing or awakening of the latent life force energy that remains

---

2   Swami Jyotirmayananda, *Concentration and Meditation* (International Yoga Society, 2013).

dormant at the base of the spine until activated by the practice of yoga. Kundalini yoga is a meditative discipline that focuses on the role of the spine, the nervous system, the chakras (energy centres) and nadis (energy channels). However, it also includes specialised breathing, asanas (postures) and meditation in awakening of this innate, primordial life force.

5. **Jnana yoga** (the yoga of wisdom) trains the intellect to become sharp and subtle. In practising jnana yoga one learns to discriminate between right and wrong, what is real and what is unreal and what is transient (changing) and what is eternal.

As mentioned earlier, yoga is a way of life and an integrated system that unites the body, mind and inner spirit. Although yoga originated in India it is universal in its applications and devoid of dogmas and demands.

One may follow any path of yoga that is suitable to one's personality. Whatever path one chooses is a matter of individual preference. The majority of people associate yoga with postures and breathing only. At the present time the followers of yoga tend to split into those who want physical benefits and those who seek a spiritual outlet. Hatha yoga, which emphasises postures (asanas), and pranayama, which focuses on breath control, constitutes only two of the eight steps of Raja yoga. The actual practice of yoga is a far more complex and integrated system of education. Yoga encompasses both the physical and spiritual aspects of being, uniting the body, mind and soul.

Practising Patanjali's eight steps of Raja yoga brings the mind under one's conscious control thus achieving inner tranquillity and enjoying lasting happiness and bliss in one's daily life. However, it must be remembered that no one path can be separated from another as they all interact with each other; movement in any path of yoga will reflect benefits in all areas. All paths of yoga lead to the same treasure-trove of making one a well-integrated and centred human being.

CHAPTER 8:

THE ESSENCE AND WISDOM OF YOGIC PHILOSOPHY: UNDERSTANDING THE SEVEN CHAKRAS, NADIS, PRANA AND KUNDALINI

W hy does yoga work? There are several reasons why yoga works. One of the basic reasons is that the ancient yogis understood the simple universal truth that the unseen, infinite, intelligent life force (prana) that is everywhere in the entire universe also exists within all human beings and all matter. Practising yoga

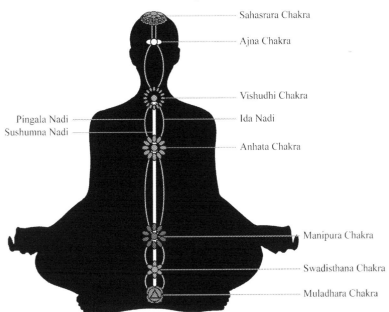

Sahasrara Chakra

Ajna Chakra

Vishudhi Chakra

Pingala Nadi
Sushumna Nadi

Ida Nadi

Anhata Chakra

Manipura Chakra

Swadisthana Chakra

Muladhara Chakra

enables us to access this unifying force of bringing the body, the mind and the soul together in a holistic manner. Since the techniques in this book are based on Kundalini yoga massage we will focus on how the concept of Kundalini has deep roots in yogic philosophy and is one of the core reasons why yoga is so effective.

Unfortunately, despite enormous strides in technology and advancements in medical sciences our overall health and well-being has not improved much in recent times. In fact, with modern excesses, a variety of chronic ailments have become commonplace. The question then is how can the practice of yoga improve our overall health and well-being? In order to further understand the reasons why yoga works and its efficacy, we need to have a basic knowledge of yogic philosophy, human anatomy and the concept of Kundalini.

The spinal column consists of thirty-three bones, called vertebrae, and these vertebrae are joined together to form the spinal column which houses the delicate spinal cord, the nerves and the cerebro spinal fluid. The spinal column acts like the trunk of a tree or an axis which supports our body's organs and structures.

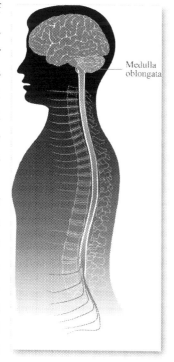

Medulla oblongata

According to yogic philosophy the life force energy present in human beings flows within subtle energy channels located in the spinal column. These subtle channels are called nadis. There are over 72,000 nadis; the main nadis are called Sushumna, Ida and Pingala. The Sushumna is the main nadi and is analogous to the spinal cord. The nadis have a tubular structure similar to a battery. In just the same way the batteries in our cell phones, tablets and iPads need to be charged regularly to function, the human body requires recharging regularly by life force energy. Along the line of the Sushumna nadi we find subtle, wheel-like energy centres called chakras. *"Chakra"* is a Sanskrit word which means "wheel." These chakras are located along the spinal column starting with the first chakra called the Muladhara. This chakra is located at the base of the spine. Each chakra controls a different function in the body. The Muladhara or base chakra is where our innate potential to live a balanced and integrated life lies dormant until activated. The seventh and the highest chakra is the Sahasrara which is located on top of the skull. It is through the practice of yoga that the Kundalini energy that lies dormant at the base of the spine is awakened and made to rise up this channel crossing each chakra until it reaches the Sahasrara chakra. The Sahasrara chakra is the reservoir for the storage of cosmic energy. If you ever experienced a heavy blow to your head and saw thousands of light flashes you will realise that this was caused by the forceful displacement of stored energy.

Anatomically the first chakra (Muladhara) and the second chakra (Swadisthana) are located in the vicinity of the sacro-coccygeal plexus whilst the third chakra (Manipura) is located in the vicinity of the solar plexus. The Muladhara chakra is extremely important in Kundalini yoga because, according to yogic philosophy, the life force energy that exists in all humans lies dormant in the vicinity of the Muladhara chakra until activated by the practice of yoga. The fourth chakra is called the heart chakra (Anahata) and is located in the area of the cardiothoracic plexus near the vicinity of the heart. The fifth chakra (Vishudda) is located in the throat area which lies in the vicinity of the carotid plexus. The sixth chakra (Ajna) is located in the centre of the forehead between the eyebrows which is in the vicinity of the medulla plexus. The area in between the eyebrows is often referred to as the third eye or spiritual eye. The seventh and final chakra (Sahasrara) is located on top of the skull which is in the vicinity of the cerebral plexus.

These chakras together with the nerves act as a giant telephone exchange where the exchange of energy occurs. This energy is then channelled to other areas via the nadis. These chakras and nadis are subtle energy centres and channels located along the length of the Sushumna nadi.

The Ida nadi begins in the right reproductive region of the perineum and crosses the Sushumna at the Muladhara chakra and again at the Anahata and Ajna chakras and then flows out through the left nostril. The Ida nadi is a moon nadi; it is cool in nature and controls the blood pressure and overflow of bile. The ida nadi is mystically described as the river Ganges and is a channel for emotional energy.

The Pingala nadi is a sun nadi and arises in the left perineum close to the reproductive area. The Pingala nadi crosses the Sushmana at the Muladhara, Anahata, and Ajna chakras and then flows out through the right nostril. The Pingala nadi, being a sun nadi, is hot in nature and regulates the digestive system. The Pingala nadi symbolically represents the Yamuna river and is a channel for intellectual energy.

The nadis are the subtle tubular columns through which life force energy flows. These energy centres (chakras) and energy channels (nadis) can be activated by the practice of asanas, pranayama, concentration and intense meditation. The science of controlling this omnipresent life force through breathing is called pranayama. Through a variety of different breathing techniques the life force energy can be accessed consciously as a vitalising, regenerative force that not only heals our bodies but also assists us in our spiritual development. Mastering the different breathing techniques enables one to access this universal life force energy to re-energise, renew and revitalise one's body, mind and spirit.

Prana is the life force energy, vital for life, and has a direct effect on the body, mind and soul. According to renowned author of *Autobiography of a Yogi*, Swami Paramahansa Yogananda, "Prana constitutes the sparks of life finer than atomic energy."

For the purpose of our discussion, we will focus on two main kinds of prana. One is the cosmic prana that is present in the universe and sustains all things, and the other is the individual prana that is present in all human beings and sustains us through our five functions. The five functions are respiration, excretion, digestion, circulation and subtle awareness of our body and breath. It must be stated that the cosmic prana and the individual prana are not only the same in quality but one continuous presence that is omnipresent. We differentiate only for the purpose of discussion.

According to yogic philosophy the medulla oblongata acts as the antenna or satellite tower that receives this life current for the distribution throughout the body. Anatomically, the medulla oblongata is located near the base of the brain stem and is part of the brain that controls functions such as respiration, heart rate, blood pressure and digestion. Ancient yogis discovered that the area around the medulla oblongata formed the entrance where the subtle, unseen life currents that pervade the universe enter human beings as individual life force energy. The medulla oblongata acts as an antenna for the reception and distribution of the universal life force energy in just the same way as a satellite dish can receive different frequencies and wave lengths to allow us to tune in to our favourite TV shows or to listen to the radio.

Anatomically, our brain is a physical organ, whilst our mind is part of the infinite, intelligence that exists everywhere. Our mind can be tuned into different frequencies and wavelengths during our different levels of consciousness. During waking, dreaming, deep sleep and meditation, we experience different states of consciousness. During sleep, our bodies are recharged unconsciously whereas during the practice of yoga, including meditation, our bodies are recharged consciously.

As mentioned earlier, "*Kundalini*" is a Sanskrit term meaning "coiled." According to yogic philosophy, this infinite, intelligent energy in human beings lies dormant at the Muladhara chakra until activated by the practice of yoga. Since this primordial energy lies at the base of the spinal column it has a direct connection to the nervous system. Kundalini yoga massage focuses on a combination of manual massage therapies releasing blocked energy stored in the energy centres and channels as well as breath work to enhance controlled breathing (pranayama). With the seven-step massage technique special attention is paid to the body-mind integration.

During Kundalini yoga massage sessions different massage techniques are employed to activate the different chakras and enhance the flow of pranic energy through the chakras and nadis.

Traditionally, yoga exercises (asanas) were used to purify the body and activate the Kundalini. However, Kundalini yoga massage is also designed to remove physiological blockages along the spinal column, unlock the innate life force that exists at the base of the spine and improve our physical health and well-being. All these benefits together also enhance our ability to deal with stress and accelerate our spiritual growth.

Uniting the body mind and soul is the basic premise and foundation on which yoga is based. The ancient yogis discovered that for humans to function as fully integrated beings it was essential to have a well-balanced nervous system that was free from disturbances. The essence and wisdom that is inherent in all forms of yoga becomes the ultimate foundation for the human being to function in a holistic way. No matter how successful we are in this material world we are all seeking to be fulfilled and live a life of purpose and I can assure you that there is no better way than yoga. Yoga is the way.

CHAPTER 9
UNIFYING THE SCIENCE OF THE WEST AND THE WISDOM OF THE EAST

The distinction between East and West in this context is based purely on geographical and cultural divisions because human beings have historically coexisted with each other and the dynamic interaction that exists between them goes back thousands of years. Eastern influences, including spirituality, have been exported to the West and Western culture, including science and technology, infiltrates the East.

Whether we come from the East or from the West, one of the greatest challenges that we face today is how to adapt to the ever-changing conditions and the environment that shapes our lives. Presently, both Easterners and Westerners rely heavily on technology for their economic and social progress. However, it is also essential for us not to let our physical needs outweigh the need to nurture our spirit. Focusing only on our physical body for our health and wellness seems short sighted. There is much wisdom in the adage which says, "Where there is a healthy mind, there is a healthy body." We are not merely physical bodies we are also holistic beings with a body, mind and soul. Human beings are extremely fortunate to possess a very highly organised, integrated brain and nervous system as well as a free will to reignite the needs of our spirits, even as we continue to harness science and technology to service our needs.

In the previous chapters we briefly outlined the nervous and muscular systems and described how these systems are intricately linked. The body, of course, has several other systems that are closely integrated and work synchronistically to keep us functioning and healthy. For the purpose of this book I specifically focus on the neuromuscular system from the point of view of Western science as well as Eastern philosophies. As we begin to examine the practice of yoga more closely we discover that it is through the practice of yoga that the nervous system becomes greatly strengthened and balanced. Whilst Western science focuses on the gross anatomy, physiology and physical aspects of the nervous system, the Eastern yogic philosophies focus on the subtle energy channels and energy centres that exist within the brain and spinal column. In yogic terminology, the cerebro spinal system consists of the Sahasradala (the brain) and the Sushumna (the spinal column).

Through a combination of various techniques such as asanas (postures), pranayama (controlling life force through specialised breathing), mental relaxation, concentration and meditation, yoga helps to rejuvenate our brain and physical body and promote healing and wellness. By practising specialised breathing techniques the blood is decarbonised and the oxygenated blood is then transmitted as life energy to revitalise the body. Through disciplined and regular practice of yoga and meditation one can start seeing the visible positive effects showing up in one's daily life. Today, there are several research studies by [1]Dr Andrew Newburg confirming the positive neurochemical and neuroelectrical effects of meditation. Yogis have developed the ability to consciously energise their

---

1   Dr. Andrew Newburg, *The Mystical Mind* (Fortress Press, 1999).

spine by controlling and distributing the flow of energy. This is achieved through intense austerities, regular practice of yoga, and self-discipline

Whether we view the body from a Western or Eastern perspective it is important to realise that all the different systems in the human body are interconnected in a perfect network; everything is continuously working day and night to manage our physical bodies. Since yoga is a discipline that unites us in a holistic way it becomes the key to accessing the healing power within all of us. Yoga focuses on the health of a person as a unified being incorporating the body, mind and soul; therefore, it surpasses all other forms of self-improvement. The techniques used in *Kundalini Yoga Massage* are also based on yogic philosophies and therefore can become the first step to assist you in your journey to total good health.

According to yogic philosophy the entire universe is seen as a manifestation of pure consciousness and human beings are a miniature representation of the universe. From a Western point of view this philosophy is equivalent to the saying "as in the macrocosm, so in the microcosm." According to Albert Einstein, "Everything in life is vibration." The body has approximately one hundred trillion cells which are made up of complex proteins, RNA, DNA and genes. These cells within our body operate and function in much the same way as the planets in our solar system. The fact that these cells lie in very close proximity to each other and are vibrating at extremely high speeds and still remain separate without colliding is a miracle. This vibrating, infinite, intelligent, universal life force (prana) that exists everywhere is responsible for all the cohesion and networking that keeps our bodies functioning and it also governs all the natural and subtler laws of the universe. From our basic knowledge in chemistry we know that everything is made up of atoms which are vibrating at a certain speed and frequency and this causes them to appear as solid, liquid or gas. Likewise, everything that we perceive or manifest in this life, including our thoughts, are associated with specific vibrations.

Our thoughts are one of the most powerful forces in the universe and they are as powerful as electromagnetic or gravitational forces. The new innovations that we see in the field of science and technology are the direct results of our evolution in thinking. Ancient yogis understood the power of thought and learnt how to tap the subtler forces that exist in the universe. There are extensive scientific studies to demonstrate how the natural laws of the universe work but there are also subtler laws that govern how the universe works which if accurately developed can have far-reaching possibilities. By combining modern science with ancient wisdom we can continue not only to excel in the field of innovation but also to improve our personal growth and self-development.

Until recently, the health benefits of yoga were based on anecdotal evidence. In more recent times with the advent of sophisticated imaging technology developed in the West there have been several research studies investigating exactly how yoga affects the human body. Evidence-based results using magnetic resonance imaging, blood tests and neurochemical and neuroelectrical tests confirm the efficacy of yoga as results can be duplicated over and over again.[2] There are several research studies that show how, through the practice of yoga, a wide variety of positive changes have been achieved.

We are lucky to be living in an exceptional period of time when, as a result of phenomenal advancement in science and modern technology, people from the West and East can exchange ideas and thoughts more freely and, nowadays, instantaneously. Whether we reside in the East or West it behoves us to look at the technology that we have created with renewed awareness and wisdom. We are not

2   Dr Herbert Benson, *The Relaxation Response.*

mechanical beings and our planet cannot survive on mechanical unity only but we can use technology as an educational tool to make better health choices and improve our overall self-development. It is extremely important for all human beings to awaken and rehabilitate the dormant life force energy that exists within all of us through the practice of yoga. By stimulating this life force energy we revitalise our body, clear our minds and increase our healing ability.

In the next chapter we will see how our fast-paced, modern lifestyle affects our nervous system and how Kundalini yoga massage can be a beneficial first step to improve not only our overall health and well-being, physically, mentally and spiritually, but also to enhance our yoga practice. By proactively unifying Western science with spiritual awareness from the East we can enrich our world far more than we ever imagined.

CHAPTER 10
THE EFFECTS OF A MODERN LIFESTYLE ON THE NERVOUS SYSTEM AND HOW YOGA AND KUNDALINI YOGA MASSAGE CAN HELP

The pace at which technology has overtaken the modern world leaves us in awe. Most of the new methods of communication are made possible because we have learnt to tap cosmic forces by mechanical means. Despite phenomenal advances in health care and technology it is sad to note that the quality of our lives as well as our overall health and well-being have not improved. It seems that in our haste to progress and keep things in our visible, material world in an orderly manner, especially in relation to time and space, we have forgotten to still our minds and gain control of our beings by accessing the inherent life force that exists within all of us. In this chapter we will focus on how stress affects us and discuss a few ways to decrease the negative effects of stress.

From the preceding chapters we learnt the nervous system is a very delicately integrated system that is responsible for every movement and function in our body, including our thoughts. In an ideal, stress-free world all the systems in a healthy individual would be working optimally.

Unfortunately, our busy modern lifestyle causes our nervous system to be constantly inundated with external stimuli that over-stimulate our emotions. The everyday stressors of work, personal life and external stimulations wear out our minds and cause our muscles to tense up instead of relaxing. Unbeknown to us, violent movies and television shows, loud music and a few other forms of "recreation" over-stimulate our nervous systems and cause a variety of stress-related symptoms.

As a result of our busy lifestyle we have come to think of relaxation as something that has to be scheduled into our daily calendar, if and when time permits. If more pressing or urgent matters usurp our time then the relaxation or quiet time is put on the back burner and the anxiety and stress continue to build up. We must learn how to prioritise our schedules to include time to heal our bodies and nurture our souls. We mentioned earlier that in this fast-paced world we are quickly becoming depersonalised, mechanical beings. We have to remind ourselves that we do not have a switch we can turn on and off at our whim, when we want to relax.

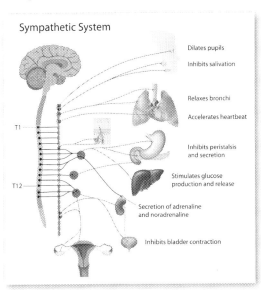

Sympathetic System

Dilates pupils

Inhibits salivation

Relaxes bronchi

Accelerates heartbeat

T1

Inhibits peristalsis and secretion

Stimulates glucose production and release

T12

Secretion of adrenaline and noradrenaline

Inhibits bladder contraction

If we are ready to make lifestyle changes to achieve a more balanced, wholesome and fulfilled life, then the practice of yoga is the answer. In the previous chapter we mentioned that the practice of yoga strengthens and balances our nervous system and through disciplined practice a variety of positive effects will start showing up in our activities of daily living. Instead of constantly expending energy and being stressed out we will become more efficient, tranquil and stress free as we begin to access the dormant life force energy that exists within us.

Earlier in the book we discussed how the sympathetic nervous system operates below the conscious level and when activated prepares us for fight or flight, mobilising our bodies to take immediate action. This system was designed as a defence mechanism by nature to be activated in times of impending danger and emergencies. Unfortunately, the stress of living in this fast-paced, modern world has caused our bodies to be in a chronic state of fight-or-flight mode. A variety of conscious and unconscious stimuli causes the sympathetic nervous system to be activated. Activation of the sympathetic nervous system leads to a series of physiological events that cause an increase in our heart and respiration rates, an increase in our blood pressure and an interference in our digestion. This causes our bodies to go into a state of dysfunction.

Moreover, it is important to realise that as we perceive the world through our five senses approaching danger, anger and anxiety all automatically stimulate the sympathetic nervous system. Suppose you are walking in the dark and see something which appears to be a snake. The sympathetic nervous system sends a message to your brain and you instinctively get prepared to run to avoid being bitten. As your body prepares for flight someone shines a light and you see that you had mistaken a coiled rope for a snake and immediately your sympathetic nervous system is deactivated. The stress of our modern-day lives keeps our body, mind and senses continually bombarded by external stimulation. Therefore, there is no chance to rejuvenate the body or the mind to achieve optimal health.

Our body can only achieve relaxation when little or no energy is consumed. Sleep is nature's way of recharging our bodies daily. Unfortunately, disease and dysfunction have become so common that millions of people have come to rely on taking medication just to enjoy a restful night's sleep. Lack of sleep can be detrimental to our health and well-being in a wide variety of ways and tends to deplete our innate life force energy. There is vast research on the subject of the deleterious effects of sleep deprivation.

We all need to rest, relax and recharge from time to time. The most common way people achieve this need is to take a vacation. However, the most obvious and common sense way to rest, relax and recharge would be to make a fundamental life style change and make a habit of daily relaxation incorporating concentration, meditation, yoga postures and simple breathing techniques. The energy and power boost and numerous other tangible benefits would be transformative. Why stop at recharging our cell phones, tablets and iPads when we can recharge ourselves daily for optimal functioning!

From the preceding chapter we know that activating our parasympathetic nervous system has the opposite effect to activating our sympathetic nervous system. The parasympathetic nervous system slows down our heart and respiration rates, lowers our blood pressure and returns our body to normal rest-and-repair mode.

There is absolutely no doubt that the negative effects of stress and other stress-related disorders have a direct adverse effect on the nervous system. From our previous discussion we know that the practice of yoga can bring balance and tranquillity to the body, mind and spirit. In this book, when we refer to the practice of yoga, we collectively mean postures, specialised breath control (pranayama), concentration and meditation. These are ancient, established techniques which help us achieve unity within ourselves and our environment.

Most of us lead busy lives and are dedicated to keeping our external world organised. We literally and figuratively don't have time to stop and smell the roses or to nurture our soul. It is time to evaluate our lives and incorporate a few simple steps to improve our health and wellbeing. I can assure you that by taking these steps you will be rewarded with high dividends.

Throughout the book, I make reference to Patanjali's eight-step guideline to better living. It is essential for the reader to understand all eight steps which are formulated to guide us to become unified and each step plays a pivotal role in this unification. For the purpose of this book, I have focused only on four of the eight steps. In chapter 7 a synopsis of the four steps are outlined. However, the four steps are so important and integral to the purpose of this book that a brief discussion of the four steps together with a discussion on *Kundalini yoga massage* is provided below.

Asanas: Although asanas are often equated with simple physical exercises we must develop a conscious awareness that asanas are slow, rhythmic stretches that are designed to promote overall health. The slow, deliberate stretching of the asanas brings flexibility to the spine, the joints and the muscles. Stretching elongates the deep holding forces of the body which includes the ligaments and tendons. In addition to bringing flexibility to the physical body the asanas focus on breath control and by revitalising the nervous system, reduce nervous disturbances and improve circulation. In addition to these physical benefits the asanas are designed to promote balance, steadiness and tranquillity of the mind. Practising the regular, slow and steady pace of the asanas also stimulates the life force energy that sits dormant at the base of the spine. Activating the release of this intelligent life force energy promotes healing, decreases the negative effect of bad habits and encourages overall integration. For those readers who wish to incorporate asanas and pranayama into their daily routines, numerous books, CDs and DVDs are available in bookstores and libraries.

Pranayama: Throughout the book, we focused on the importance of pranayama (specialised breath control). It is a well-known fact that human beings can survive without food or water for a short period of time but it is impossible for anyone to survive without breathing. Learning how to focus the mind on the flow of the breath may appear to be a simple technique but I can assure you that it will have a far-reaching effect in your journey to optimal health and self-realisation. The science of correct breathing is the clearest index of our inner consciousness. Disturbances in our mind are signalled by disturbances in our breathing.

Through the disciplined and regular practice of yoga we can gain control of our breath and, in turn, we can control our life force energy. In yoga, prana is the subtle, life-giving energy that exists in the universe which we can access through controlled breathing. The practice of pranayama strengthens the respiratory system and the organs associated with it. The yogis learnt to transcend their senses and through disciplined practice they have attained mastery over controlling the flow of prana. However, these techniques are not only to be used by saints and sages as we all have an innate, intelligent life force lying dormant within us.

Millions of ordinary people who practice regular and disciplined yoga have come to understand and appreciate how yoga not only improved their health and well-being but was also beneficial in all other areas of their lives. Throughout the book I have made the readers aware that our breath is an outward manifestation of the flow of prana that exists everywhere in the universe and within humans as well. The breath is the switch that controls our engine which is our body and by gaining control of the switch we gain control of our body. In Chapter 11, at the end of session four, this book focuses on a few simple pranayama techniques. For more complex techniques it is necessary to get guidance from a professional yoga instructor.

Concentration and Meditation: Another way to tap into the universal life force is through the regular practice of concentration and meditation. Concentration is the act of training the mind to concentrate on one point or idea. During concentration you may focus your mind on a concrete form, for example, the flame of a candle or you may focus on a symbol such as AUM. Concentration allows the mind to move from a state of being dull and distracted to a state of one pointedness and control. The one pointed mind is free from the numerous distractions of daily living that so dominate our minds and also free from the pressure of the negative impressions of the subconscious mind. As the pressures of the day are often overwhelming it takes repeated, on-going effort to achieve the goal of one pointedness. It is natural for the mind to flit from one thought to another. Self-observation and self-awareness are absolutely essential in the effort to achieve one pointedness.

Meditation: Meditation is a state of consciousness when our thought waves are stilled consciously for a long period of time and the mind is turned inward. During meditation the heart rate, pulse rate and blood pressure are all lowered and breathing becomes slow and deep. The reception of life force energy increases and the cells of the body are recharged, rejuvenated and repaired. During meditation we try to stop our thoughts consciously whilst during sleep we stop our thoughts unconsciously. In this way through the regular, disciplined practice of pranayama and meditation our sympathetic nervous system and stress responses are deactivated whilst the parasympathetic nervous system and relaxation responses are activated. Meditation is essential for developing our inner faculties; in our daily routine this may be seen as a system of checks and balances to evaluate our lives. Today, most people spend an enormous amount of time improving their outer physical bodies but tend to neglect their inner being. The science of meditation provides the mind with a favourable environment and nourishment for reaching the highest potential of growth, both physically and spiritually. There are various forms of meditative techniques and the readers can chose whatever technique they wish, as long as it suits their personality. Information on meditation is widely available. I strongly urge readers to make a commitment to include meditation as part of their daily routine and they will be pleasantly surprised with the positive changes that will start to manifest in their lives.

Kundalini yoga massage: Our bodies are continuously subjected to the negative effects of internal and external stimulation causing enormous stress. Kundalini yoga massage is based on sound yogic principles and becomes the first step to promote healing of body, mind and soul.

Kundalini yoga massage techniques are designed to take you from stress to serenity. The aim of the techniques outlined in this book is to remove physiological blockages that can impede our quest to achieve good health. Our physical bodies are subjected to injury, stress, anxiety and fear, all of which directly affect our neuromuscular system and cause physiological blockages. Once those blockages are removed we can establish harmony and tranquillity between our physical bodies and all aspects of our being and live a more integrated life. The seven steps focus on stimulating the paraspinal soft tissue areas around the individual chakras and this assists in removing blockages and increasing the flow of prana. Whereas some yoga asanas focus on the gross movements of the spine to stimulate the flow of life force energy, Kundalini yoga massage focuses on increasing the flow of pranic energy at a much subtler level. One of the Kundalini yoga massage techniques pays special attention to the chest and rib cage areas by releasing blockages from the heart chakra. Releasing blockages from this area notably improves circulation and relaxes the rib cage, intercostal muscles and the area around the diaphragm, thereby improving our breathing. Controlled breathing exercises help eliminate carbon dioxide and toxins and this increases the supply of oxygen, encourages the flow of prana and revitalises, relaxes and nourishes the whole body.

We are all seeking to be in a state of peace. This quote from Desiderata sums it up perfectly: "Go placidly amidst the noise and the haste and remember what peace there may be in silence." I use the following formula to remind me to get into a state of peace:

$$-\overline{n} + \overline{\varsigma} = \boldsymbol{\mathcal{E}}^3$$

- N (subtract [or remove] noise and external stimulation)
+ S (add silence)
= E^3 (equates to accessing energy existing everywhere)

The primary aim of yoga is to promote a system of self-development within an individual and encourage total integration of body, mind and soul. Asanas, pranayama, concentration and meditation, and seven-step *Kundalini Yoga Massage* are important methods to achieving this integration. During the practice of yoga, we can access different levels of consciousness bringing us serenity and tranquillity which are then carried over to our activities of daily living.

In our very busy, stress-filled lives we are always looking for new and innovative ways to reduce our stressors and what better way than to combine the two very powerful techniques of Kundalini yoga and massage? As with yoga, Kundalini yoga massage will deactivate our sympathetic nervous system, activate our parasympathetic nervous system, and bring our body to a state of complete integration, returning us to the rest-and-repair mode.

Kundalini yoga massage is an important tool not only to improve and access the flow of intelligent life force present within us but also to assist in uniting our body, mind and soul, thereby enhancing our health and well-being.

Chapter 11 provides step-by-step instructions of several different massage techniques used in Kundalini yoga massage. These techniques are not meant to be used exclusively by registered massage therapists or holistic practitioners. They have been designed and formulated to be used by the general public and all avid yoga practitioners. However, I must emphasise that anyone who wishes to use Kundalini yoga massage professionally should get the proper clinical and practical training and become certified. If you only wish to use the seven-step techniques for personal use a weekend course to familiarise yourself with the basic techniques is recommended.

SUMMARY OF TYPES OF MASSAGE USED IN SEVEN-STEP TECHNIQUES

Kundalini yoga massage is a seven-step series of one-hour sessions to activate by physiological means the subtle flow of life force energy (prana) within the seven chakras.

Prior to outlining the seven steps, I will give a brief description of the various massage techniques that will be used.

ABDOMINAL MASSAGE

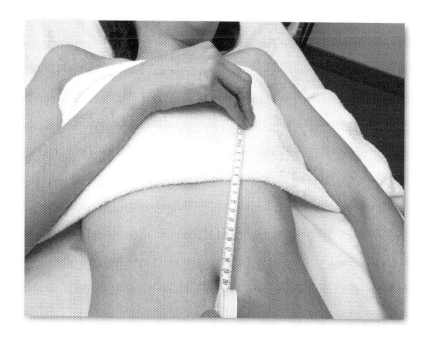

Abdominal massage begins with measuring the distance from the navel to the right nipple and then to the left nipple. This measurement is taken on the diagonal. Discrepancy in the measurement from left to right shows a misalignment of the solar plexus and is indicative of postural distortions.

Massage begins with a standard effleurage (see subsequent page) warm-up, using the palmar aspects of both hands. Your hands should move in a clockwise direction (the same direction in which digestion takes place). Start under the rib cage and proceed in a clockwise direction using circular motions. Continue with clockwise massage for seven to eleven repetitions or until navel-to-nipple alignment is restored. Always restore alignment in the solar plexus before proceeding with subsequent steps.

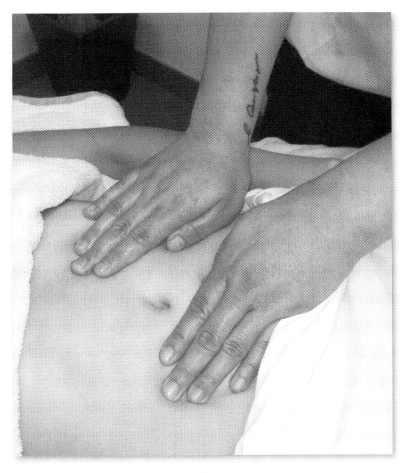

ACUPRESSURE

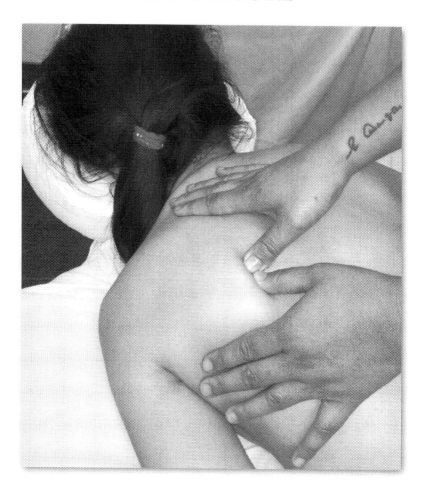

Physical pressure using the hand or elbow will be applied in certain areas to release tension and improve the flow of life force energy.

CRISS-CROSS FIBRE FRICTION

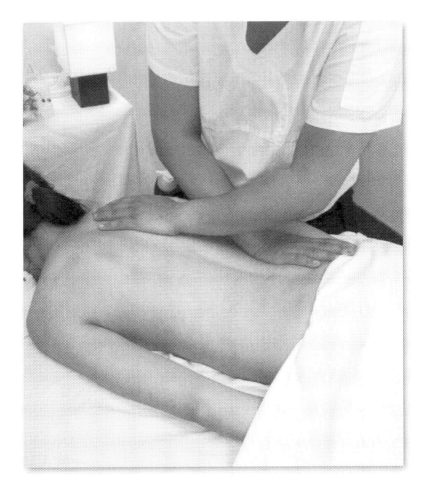

Criss-cross fibre friction uses the palm of the hand or the fingers. The force comes from the heel of the hand or from the fingers. A deep, firm, circular motion to break down scar tissue and improve circulation is used.

DEEP TISSUE MASSAGE

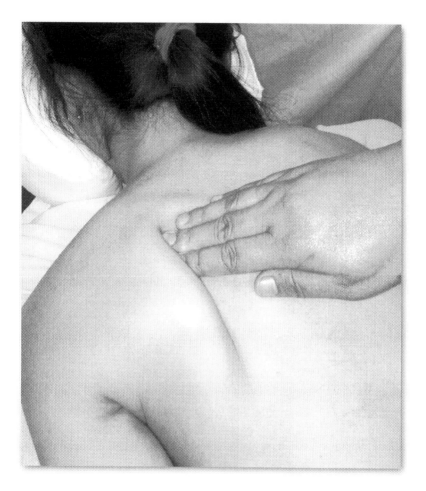

This technique focuses on muscles located below the surface including the connective tissue and fascia. Deep tissue massage helps relieve tension in the muscles and can be applied to both superficial and deep layers. Deep tissue massage can be performed using the palm, elbow or fingers. When using the heel of the hand glide from side to side.

EFFLEURAGE

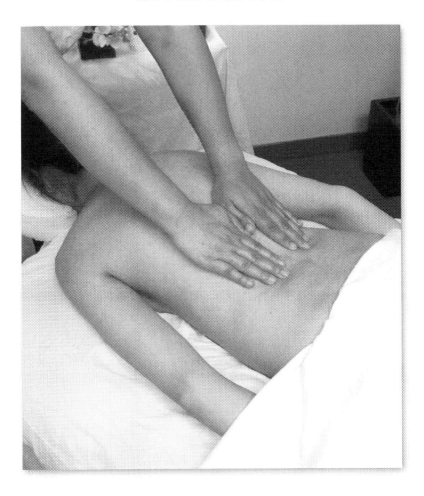

Effleurage can be a gentle or a firm massage using stroking, sliding or gliding to warm up muscles. Stroking movements are performed using the palm of the hands. This technique warms up muscles and also encourages increased circulation and lymphatic drainage.

FACE AND HEAD MASSAGE

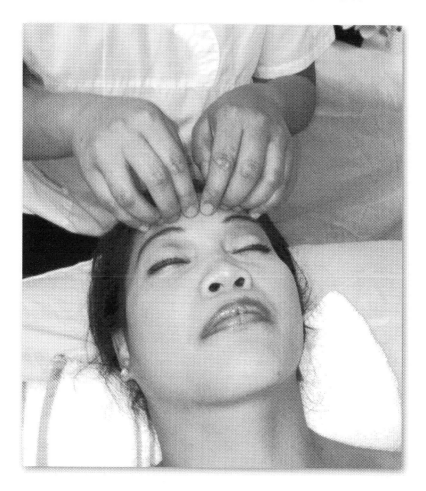

For the entire face including the frontal sinus area a combination of effleurage, acupressure, gentle tapping and vibration massage is used. Rejuvenating face massage opens up blockages in the area of the sixth chakra and improves the flow of prana. The head massage is performed with the palm of both hands. The fingers and thumbs are also used with gentle, light stroking movements. Gentle tapping and vibration massage are used for the top of the skull. The head massage is finished by making small circles all over the scalp area. For the base of the head trigger point therapy is effective in improving the flow of the lymphatic system and life force energy.

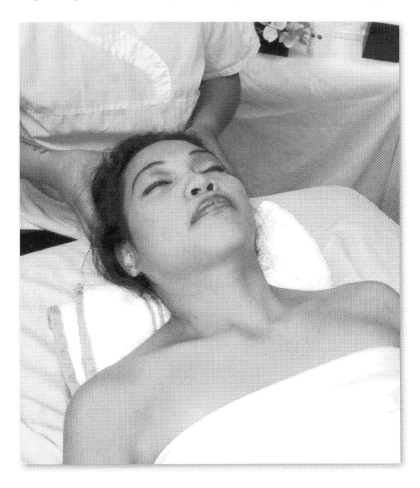

KNEADING

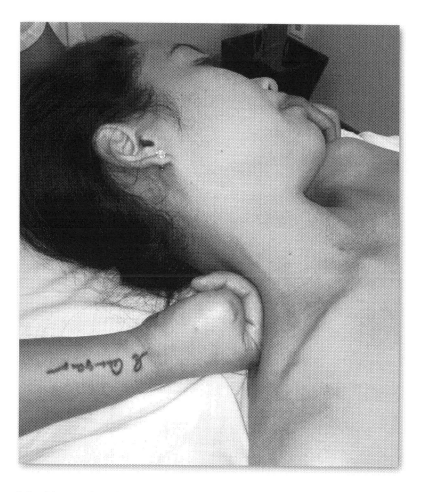

Mould your hands into a closed fist and gently press your fist into the muscles.

PETRISSAGE

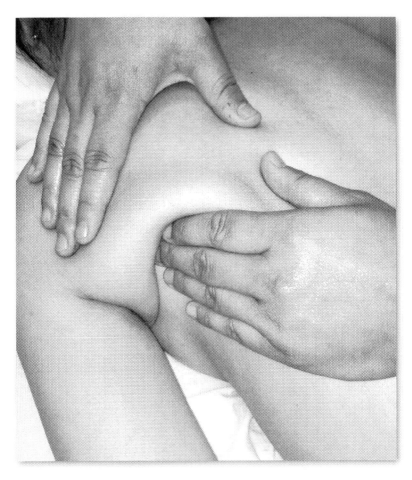

Movements are done with either the palmar aspect of the hand or fingers and thumbs. Massage movements are applied with enough pressure to compress underlying muscles. Petrissage combines several different massage techniques that include kneading, pick and squeeze, wringing, skin rolling, pinching and stretching. During the course of Kundalini yoga massage a combination of several techniques will be used to activate the energy centres (chakras) and the energy channels (nadis), thereby releasing physiological blockages.

SACRAL PUMP

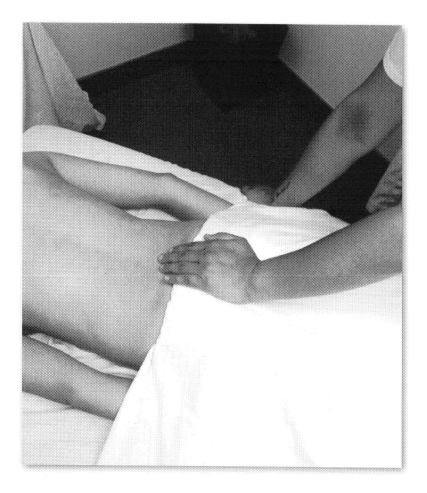

Mould your hand into a cup shape and place the palm of your hand over the sacral coccygeal area. Gently mobilise the sacrum back and forth to activate the first and second chakras. This is a vital step in Kundalini yoga massage. According to yogic philosophy our latent life force energy lies dormant in this area until activated.

SCISSORING

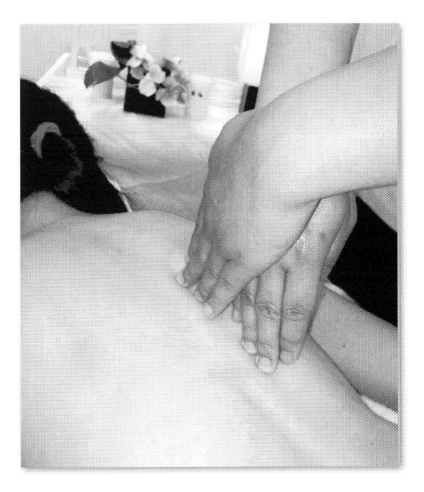

Scissoring is another petrissage technique. The index and middle fingers of both hands are used. The hands are placed opposite each other and slowly worked away from each other by lifting and releasing.

TAPPING/CUPPING

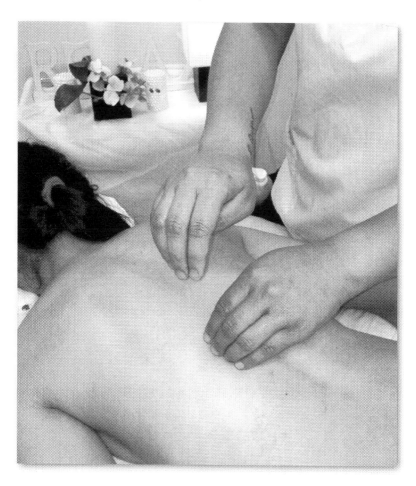

This technique is a rhythmic percussion using the cupped hand or fingertips. Hands are moulded into a cup-like shape and the muscles are gently tapped rhythmically. This technique is effective for stimulating the nervous and lymphatic systems and releasing the blocked energy centres.

TRIGGER POINT THERAPY

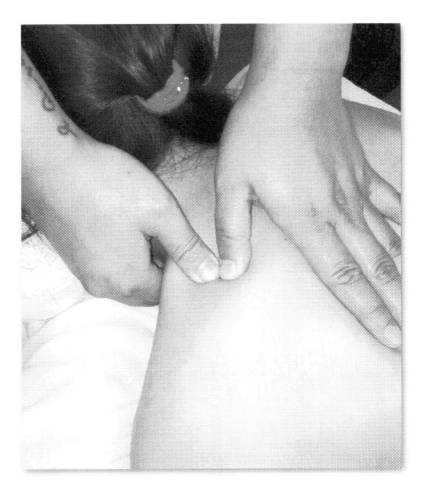

Manual pressure is applied to areas that cause local pain or referred pain. Trigger points relate to dysfunction in the neuromuscular junction. Trigger point therapy is essential in Kundalini yoga massage because it assists in removing blockages from the neuromuscular junctions and improves the flow of prana from the chakras and nadis.

VIBRATION/SHAKING

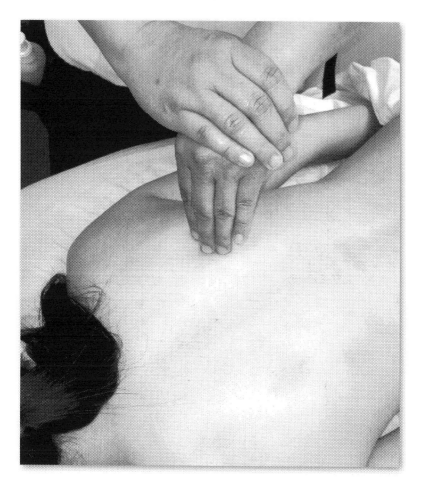

The fingers or palm of the hand are used. The intensity goes from medium to strong. Vibrations should be performed rhythmically.

CHAPTER 11
SEVEN-STEP TECHNIQUES TO PERFORM KUNDALINI YOGA MASSAGE

Kundalini yoga massage is a seven-step series of one-hour sessions to activate the subtle flow of energy (prana) by physiological means. Kundalini yoga massage is a combination of several manual massage therapy techniques to remove physiological blockages from the energy centres and breath work to enhance controlled breathing (pranayama). It also encourages body-mind integration by focusing on stress self-awareness which allows us to become conscious of how stress affects us both physically and mentally. "The mind acts on the body and the body acts on the mind. Every mental state creates a corresponding state in the body and every action in the body has a corresponding effect on the mind."[1] These wise words spoken by Swami Vivekananda in 1900 still hold true today.

1   Swami Vivekananda, "Powers of the Mind, Eighth Impression." Delivered at Los Angeles, California, January 8, 1900.

SESSION 1

ONE-HOUR SESSION
CHAKRAS 1 AND 2 (MULADHARA AND SWADISTHANA)
LOCATED IN THE VICINITY OF
SACRO-COCCYGEAL PLEXUS

(includes completing patient history and consent forms, biomechanical and gait analysis forms)

THIRTY MINUTES OF FIRST SESSION

In order to evaluate treatment outcomes and to monitor the efficacy of the treatment the therapist should conduct a systematic, step-by-step patient evaluation. The goal of the first session is for the patient and practitioner to familiarise themselves with each other. Thirty minutes of the first session are spent on history taking and medical data collection as well as a detailed biomechanical and gait analysis.

1. A detailed patient history is collected including physical examination and laboratory reports.
2. A detailed gait analysis and biomechanical evaluation must be conducted by the therapist. This is to assist in gaining maximum benefits.
3. Any specific problems must be identified and any impairments in function (be it physical, psychological, social or vocational) resulting from disease or secondary impairment must be documented.
4. Once all the data has been collected and evaluated a specific treatment plan will be customised for each patient in keeping with the guidelines of seven-step Kundalini yoga massage.

5. Customisations will take into account the general state of patients' health, their age and their ability to lie either prone or supine for a prolonged length of time.

6. During each session progress notes must be accurately recorded and subsequent changes to the treatment plan must also be documented.

    Attachments: 1. Patient Consent Form
                   2. Patient History Form and Progress Notes
                   3. Biomechanical and Gait Analysis Forms
                   4. Patient Feedback Form

7. Any previous experiences with yoga, yogic philosophy or meditation are also documented.

8. Any previous knowledge of yoga or yogic philosophy will enhance the benefits of Kundalini yoga massage.

9. A physical examination of the patient's spine and paraspinal areas is performed.

10. At this stage the patient's spinal range of motion is evaluated and recorded.

11. The goal of the first session is for the patient and practitioner to familiarise themselves with each other and gain a clear understanding of the patient's health concerns.

12. It is important to understand what the patient's expectations are.

13. Once the history has been completed and the data collection recorded the therapist should ensure that the physical surroundings have been set up to promote tranquillity and serenity. It is also important for the patient to be relaxed both mentally and physically.

14. The practitioner can take a few minutes to verbally assist the patient with progressive relaxation, from head to toe.

15. Seven-step Kundalini yoga massage is a manual therapy designed to remove any physiological blockages from the vicinity of the seven chakras. Kundalini yoga massage also activates the life force energy that lies dormant at the base of the spine and sets in motion a series of physiological events that promote healing.

Please note: It is essential to include steps 9 through 15 in all seven steps of Kundalini yoga massage as it is our aim to activate the subtle energy centres (chakras) and energy channels (nadis), to remove physiological blockages and to encourage the flow of life force energy.

At the very end of each session with the patient lying in the prone position a few minutes must be spent on stimulating the paraspinal muscles on the right and left side of the spine. Begin the massage from the base of the spine and continue to the base of the skull. The techniques used here can be a combination of petrissage and effleurage. This ensures that the chakras and nadis have been activated, encouraging the flow of life force energy. To ensure the flow of pranic energy via the front of the forehead and the top of the skull a minute or two is spent on the patient to perform the techniques outlined for the face and head massage.

Although the massage techniques are designed to remove physical blockages it is important for both the practitioner and patient to realise that stimulating the chakras activates a series of physiological changes within the body that will become the beneficial foundation to heal not just the body but the mind and soul.

SECOND HALF OF FIRST SESSION

1. The patient is placed prone on the massage table.
2. This session focuses on the first and second chakras.
3. During this session the areas in and around the sacro-coccygeal plexus are addressed.
4. Both the fascia and soft tissue at the base of the spine are warmed by gentle massaging for ten minutes.
5. Moist hot packs may be used to assist in warming this area.
6. The soft tissue structures are then stretched and elongated to break down any adhesions present.
7. Once the area is warmed up gentle pressure gradually builds up to deeper pressure.
8. It is important for the practitioner to communicate regularly with the patient in order to develop a bearable tolerance to the pressure applied during the massage.
9. A combination of different massage techniques is used to stimulate the area. These techniques include kneading, wringing, skin rolling, finger rolling, pick and squeeze technique, acupressure and the sacral pump.
10. These techniques are performed using the palmar aspect of the hand as well as the fingers and thumbs.
11. All movements are slow and rhythmical and administered in the paraspinal area in close proximity to sacro-coccygeal area.
12. Scissoring (criss-cross stretching) is also applied.
13. The middle and index fingers of the hand are placed opposite each other and slowly worked away from each other lifting and releasing as you go.
14. A combination of all these techniques lasts approximately twenty-five minutes.

THE FINAL FIVE MINUTES OF SESSION 1

1. The last five minutes are spent on the sacral pump. The palm of the hand is placed over the sacrum and coccyx and the sacrum is then mobilised back and forth to activate the first and second chakra and release the flow of prana.

Note: All massage therapy techniques in all sessions focus on soft tissue mobilisation. The soft tissue includes the fascia, the skeletal muscles and the holding forces.

SESSION 2
ONE-HOUR SESSION
THIRD CHAKRA (MANIPURA)
IN THE VICINITY OF THE SOLAR PLEXUS

Please note that the patient must be instructed to refrain from eating two to three hours prior to the massage treatment. If the patient is experiencing diarrhoea or loose bowel movements then abdominal massage is contra indicated. The first thirty minutes are spent in repeating techniques in Session 1. The second thirty minutes focus on the third chakra.

FIRST THIRTY MINUTES OF SESSION 2

1. The patient lies prone for the first thirty-minute session.
2. Progress notes are recorded.
3. Any discomfort or side effects must be documented.
4. This session begins with a moist hot pack applied to the thoracolumbar and sacral area for ten minutes.

5. It is easier to mobilise the soft tissue when the muscles and fascia are warm and pliable.

6. Once the hot pack has been removed, five minutes are spent in the sacro-coccygeal area and a combination of techniques used in Session 1 is applied.

7. The sacral pump technique is also included.

8. A combination of the same techniques of kneading, skin rolling, finger rolling, wringing, pick and squeeze and acupressure are applied to the paraspinal area in line with the thoracolumbar area.

9. These techniques assist in relaxing the muscles and fascia in this area.

SECOND THIRTY MINUTES OF SESSION 2

1. The third chakra is located in the vicinity of the navel.

2. During the second thirty-minute session the patient lies supine.

3. The second thirty minutes are focused on a specialised massage to the abdominal area to ensure the proper alignment of the solar plexus.

4. Prior to the abdominal massage a measurement is taken from the navel to the left nipple of the breast diagonally and this measurement is recorded.

5. This is followed by taking a measurement diagonally from the navel to the right nipple and this measurement is also recorded.

6. If there is a discrepancy in the measurements then there is a misalignment of the abdominal muscles and postural distortions are present.

7. Begin using effleurage technique to massage the abdominal muscles clockwise in a circular direction.

8. The massage is administered using the palmar aspect of the hand.
9. Start under the rib cage area of one side and proceed in a clockwise direction to the other side using circular motions.
10. This circular movement is repeated seven to eleven times (or longer) until alignment is achieved.
11. The navel-to-nipple measurement is taken once again until both the measurements are equal.
12. This indicates that all postural distortions have been removed and the abdominal muscles and the solar plexus are now aligned.
13. The abdominal massage helps stimulate the deeper abdominal muscles and may facilitate bowel movements.
14. Hence, care should be taken to apply moderate pressure that is tolerable for the patient.
15. The abdominal area is considered the core of the body and much of the body's energy is transferred through the core.
16. The abdominal massage is effective in aligning the solar plexus and releases tension associated with the internal organs.
17. This is a very powerful and effective method; massaging along the lines of the energy channels of the body helps to balance the right and left side of the body.
18. All blocked energy (prana) is now able to flow freely.
19. With the proper alignment of the body the patient experiences deep relaxation and a sense of well-being in all areas: physical, spiritual, emotional and mental.
20. The patient who meditates will experience a deeper more intense state of relaxation.

SESSION 3
ONE-HOUR SESSION
REVIEW SESSION

Patient lies prone for most of this session except for a brief period when the abdominal massage is being performed. This entire one-hour session focuses on repeating the techniques for the first, second and third chakras as in Sessions 1 and 2.

SESSION 4
ONE-HOUR SESSION
FOURTH CHAKRA (ANAHATA OR HEART CHAKRA)
IN THE VICINITY OF THE CARDIAC PLEXUS

This session focuses on the heart chakra which is located in the cardiothoracic area.

FIRST THIRTY MINUTES OF SESSION 4

1. The first thirty minutes of Session 4 focus on repeating the techniques of the first, second and third chakras.

SECOND THIRTY MINUTES OF SESSION 4

1. This session focuses on releasing the prana in the Anahata (heart) chakra which is the fourth chakra. Patient lies prone for most of this session.
2. This chakra is located in the cardiac region.
3. For five minutes of the second thirty minutes the patient is covered with a moist hot pack in the cardiothoracic region.

4. The next ten minutes are dedicated to the paraspinal muscles in the cardiothoracic area.
5. Once again, the same techniques of kneading, skin rolling, finger rolling, pick and squeeze and acupressure are applied in the paraspinal area opposite the fourth chakra.
6. In this way the muscles that are found in the cardiac area in the vicinity of the fourth chakra are stimulated.
7. The next five minutes are spent working on the back of the rib cage as this assists in loosening and relaxing the intercostal muscles.

THIRD TEN MINUTES OF SESSION 4

The patient lies supine for the last ten minutes of this session.

1. The last ten minutes of this session are allocated to massaging the anterior intercostal area of the rib cage and the anterior cardiothoracic area is addressed.
2. Special attention is focused on the area below the diaphragm.
3. Extra care should be taken when massaging these areas as many delicate organs are located in this area.
4. A combination of effleurage and long stroking technique is used for the anterior rib cage area.
5. This technique will allow any adhesions in the intercostal area to be broken down.
6. Before the end of this session patients are encouraged to breathe using their entire torso.
7. This is natural, rhythmical breathing and involves the use of the abdominal area and a conscious effort.
8. Our everyday breathing is shallow and left to the control of the body's autonomic reflex system and the unconscious mind.

9. A yogic breath is a complete breath; all the stale air is forced out of the lungs prior to fresh air being drawn in.
10. This session encourages patients to develop an awareness of abdominal breathing.
11. Patients should be taught to place their hands on their chest and abdomen in order to check for correct deep breathing movements.
12. If both hands move during inhalation and exhalation then the patients are breathing correctly using their whole torso.
13. If the patient's hands do not move sufficiently during inhalation and exhalation and there is no visible movement of the diaphragm then the patient is not breathing correctly.
14. A minute or two prior to the end of the session the patient is asked to sit up and take a complete yogic breath.
15. For beginners, a typical breathing exercise as listed in (2) below will suffice.

YOGIC BREATHING TECHNIQUES
(PRANAYAMA EXERCISES)

The science of pranayama focuses on controlling the universal life force through a series of specialised breathing exercises. There are a variety of pranayama exercises. Below is a list of a few of the techniques to practice yogic breathing. Feel free to practice whichever technique you are comfortable with.

1. Breathe in for a count of three and breathe out for a count of six, the exhalation being twice as long as the inhalation as this encourages the stale air to be eliminated. The exhalation can be done to a sound of "HA."
2. If patients have difficulty exhaling their breath for a count of six then a simple pattern of breathing in for a count of

three, holding for a count of three and exhaling for a count of three can be used.

3. Another important pranayama technique is alternate nostril breathing. To begin, use your right thumb to block the right nostril and inhale through your left nostril to a count of four; then use your ring finger to close the left nostril and retain your breath to a count of sixteen; then remove your right thumb from your right nostril and exhale to a count of eight. Repeat the technique blocking the left nostril. Beginners can reduce their ratio count to 1:4:2 instead of 4:16:8. As you gain more experience you can increase the ratio by multiples of 2.

4. The classical pattern of yogic breathing is (1-4-2-4). The patient inhales for a count of one, holds for a count of four exhales for a count of two and the breath is held out for a count of four. This ratio of breathing can be increased gradually by multiples of 2, 4, 6, and so on. This type of breathing is very intense and should be done under the supervision of a highly trained yoga teacher.

5. For this yoga massage session a simple deep abdominal breathing as outlined in (2) above is sufficient.

Please note: A complete yogic breath entails inhaling slowly to completely fill the abdomen, chest and rib cage area; there is a visible movement of the diaphragm. The exhalation is twice as long as the inhalation to encourage the stale air to be eliminated completely.

SESSION 5
ONE-HOUR SESSION
FIFTH CHAKRA (VISHUDDA OR THROAT CHAKRA)

First Thirty Minutes of Session 5

1. The patient lies mostly prone during this half of the session.
2. The first ten minutes the patient is given a hot moist pack to make the muscles warm, pliable and easier to work with.
3. Note the moist pack is applied for five minutes to the thoracolumbar area and is moved up for the next five minutes to the cervical area.
4. Hot packs that are elongated can be wrapped around the throat area.
5. This ensures that both the posterior and anterior muscles in the neck and throat area are warmed up and pliable.
6. The next twenty minutes of the fifth session are spent on repeating the areas addressed in Sessions 1, 2, 3 and 4.
7. Patient feedback and progress is documented before and after each session.

SECOND THIRTY MINUTES OF SESSION 5

1. After the first thirty minutes the patient is turned to the supine position.
2. When the patient turns around the alignment of the solar plexus is measured to check if there is a discrepancy.
3. In the event of a discrepancy three to four clockwise effleurage massages should be performed (as in Session 2). This should be sufficient to restore alignment of the solar plexus. In the event that alignment is still not restored it

may be necessary to do a few more clockwise effleurage massages.

4. Next, the lateral cervical muscles on the right and left sides are massaged using criss-cross stretching, finger sliding and trigger point therapy for twenty-five minutes.

5. The patient's left and right temporomandibular (TM) joints should be examined to look for any restrictions as this will cause dysfunction in the neck and throat area.

6. If any restrictions are present the patient's TM joints and the muscles around them should be mobilised internally and externally.

7. For internal mobilisation patients are asked to open their mouth widely and the practitioner uses a gloved hand to manually mobilise the muscles on both right and left TM joints. The muscles on the outside of the joint can also be mobilised externally.

8. After the mobilisation patients are then asked to open and close their jaw to evaluate whether the TM joints are moving synchronistically.

9. The last five minutes are spent in massaging the anterior aspect of the neck; the patient is asked to take a few deep breaths in and out to remove any restrictions in the throat area as this is the location of the fifth chakra. The exhalation breath can be done to the sound "HA."

10. Once all the above techniques have been administered the life force energy (prana) will flow more easily as all restrictions will have been physiologically removed.

SESSION 6

ONE-HOUR SESSION
SIXTH AND SEVENTH CHAKRAS (AJNA AND SAHASRARA CHAKRAS) IN THE VICINITY OF THE MEDULLA PLEXUS AND CRANIAL PLEXUS

FIRST THIRTY MINUTES OF SESSION 6

1. The patient is given a hot moist pack for the first ten minutes.
2. The next twenty minutes of this session are spent on repeating the techniques outlined in Sessions 1 through 5.

SECOND THIRTY MINUTES OF SESSION 6

1. The sixth chakra is called the Ajna chakra. It is located on the forehead in between the eyes.
2. The seventh chakra is called the Sahasrara. This chakra is located on top of the skull.
3. This massage session focuses on the face, the head and the skull. The massage is initially done with the patient lying supine.
4. The face and head massage are performed without the use of creams and oils (unless the patient requests that a lubricant be used).
5. Kundalini yoga massage focuses on the area of the forehead in between the eyes as this is where the sixth chakra is anatomically located.
6. The frontal sinus area is massaged to release any blockages caused as a result of sinusitis or thickening of the mucosa.
7. A combination of effleurage, acupressure, gentle tapping and vibration massage is used in this area.

8. The entire skull is massaged using long stroking movements and special focus is directed to the top of the skull where the seventh chakra is anatomically located.

9. Particular attention is also placed on the base of the skull. This is the area where the medulla oblongata is located. As stated earlier, according to yogic philosophy, the medulla oblongata acts as an antenna that draws in the universal life force energy. Releasing any blockages from the face and skull areas is essential to improving an individual's flow of life force energy. For the base of the skull trigger point therapy is effective to help improve the flow of the lymphatic system and life force energy.

10. For the rest of the skull gentle tapping, vibration massage, stroking and trigger point techniques are used.

11. The practitioner's hands are placed on either side of the head with both thumbs on the centre of the skull. Pressure is then applied along the length of the central suture of the skull.

12. The head massage is finished by making small circles all over the scalp area.

13. For the neck area make a small fist and gently massage the side of the neck. Long, gentle stroking movements and effleurage can be used for the front of the neck and throat area.

14. Blocked energy can be caused by a variety of ailments including stress-related headaches, eye strain, tinnitus, sinusitis, insomnia and other physical organic dysfunctions.

15. Massaging the head and face removes any blockages and improves the flow of prana in the nadis (channels) and chakras (energy centres).

16. Gentle traction is applied to the base of the neck to assist in the flow of prana.

Note: At the end of Session 6 the patient is given a patient feedback evaluation form to complete and return to the practitioner on the next visit. The patient feedback evaluation form evaluates the practitioner, the techniques as well as the environment.

SESSION 7
ONE-HOUR SESSION
INCLUDES THE FIRST THROUGH
SEVENTH CHAKRAS
COVERS ALL CHAKRAS AND PLEXUSES

1. This is the seventh and final session of the series of seven one-hour Kundalini yoga massage sessions to activate the seven chakras.

2. The first ten minutes of Session 7 should focus on getting feedback from the patient.

3. The patient feedback form should be given to the patient at the end of the sixth session so that the patient has time to evaluate the questions and provide an appropriate performance rating.

4. During this period the practitioner can ask for suggestions to make the environment or surroundings more therapeutic or any other suggestions on improving treatments.

5. During the initial intake in Session 1, a biomechanical gait analysis and a full physical examination was done. In Session 7, a follow-up comparison biomechanical gait analysis and physical examination should be done.

6. This will reveal any objective benefits of the Kundalini yoga massage session. For example, results may show an overall

increase in range of motion in a particular area. We then deduce that the patient's flexibility has improved.

7.   The next fifty minutes are spent on repeating Sessions 1 to 6.

Please note: The minimum requirement for Kundalini yoga massage is seven one-hour sessions spread over a seven-week period. However, every individual responds differently to any form of physical therapy and this includes massage therapy. It is our recommendation that the therapy be customised for all patients depending on their state of health, age, fitness level and motivation. Some patients may require longer sessions or more sessions to get maximum benefits whilst seven one-hour sessions may be adequate for others.

WARNING

CONTRA INDICATIONS

Kundalini yoga massage therapy may be contra indicated for certain conditions. Please consult with your primary health care practitioner before scheduling any appointment. The author of this book is in no way responsible for the misuse of any of the techniques. It is recommended that the massage be administered by someone who has been professionally trained in these techniques.

RECOMMENDATIONS

In order to enjoy the full benefits of Kundalini yoga massage it is imperative to join a yoga studio or class that offers a complete yoga programme including asanas (postures), pranayama (controlled breathing) and meditation. In order to retain and extend the beneficial effects of Kundalini yoga massage a one-hour maintenance massage is recommended every four to six weeks. All aspects and techniques in the seven steps have been thoroughly tested and the benefits are enormous. I have attempted to outline the techniques in an easy-to-follow, step-by-step manner. I have also included photos, prints of yoga chakras and diagrams of the nervous system and the muscular system to enhance your understanding visually.

CONCLUSION

It is heart warming to note that as the practice of yoga, including meditation, is demystified more and more doctors are recommending yoga, meditation and massage to control pain and stress-related illness. Today, yoga in some form or another is being practised by millions of people worldwide simply because they have discovered and experienced first-hand its palpable benefits.

With the advancement of technology we seem to have a manual on how to operate everything from our day-to-day appliances to our cars and other machines. Unfortunately, we have not yet found a manual on how to operate human beings and it seems that all our life lessons are learnt through the obstacles and challenges that we face. We are, of course, living, breathing human beings and as soon as we stop breathing we stop living. Whilst we are living and breathing we have challenges to face and stressors to deal with and we are constantly looking for new and innovative ways to reduce our stress. Stress reduction through the practice of yoga, meditation and massage is well established. By combining yoga and massage the benefits of controlling stress are abundantly enhanced.

In the earlier chapters we likened the human body to a battery. In much the same way as electricity flows through a battery by activating the chakras we can increase the flow of life force energy (prana) for our overall well-being. This benefit encompasses all aspects of our being including the physical, emotional and spiritual elements. When energy is blocked our health and well-being is compromised.

Throughout the book I focused on prana and pranayama (specialised breathing) and how they can assist us to function as integrated beings, uniting the body, mind and soul. We have discussed at length the subtle, unseen prana which is the essence that gives the breath of life to our body. Our breath, as we know it, is just a manifestation of this unseen life force that exists everywhere. Have you ever seen the electromagnetic waves that transmit signals to your television sets, radios and cell phones? We turn on our television and magically get a clear and pristine image on our screen. Although we cannot see the electromagnetic waves we do not doubt their existence. If the signals are interrupted we get a blurred image. Unseen pranic energy works in much the same way as unseen electromagnetic waves. Dysfunction and disturbances in the nervous system impede the flow of prana (life force) in human beings.

The point that I am trying to make here is that although we cannot see the universal, infinite, intelligent life force it exists and plays a pivotal role in our existence. Therefore, if the flow of prana in an individual is uninterrupted we get a healthy, well-balanced individual and when it is impeded disease sets in.

The practice of yoga and regular massage sessions gives us respite from our daily, humdrum routine. The efficacy of yoga to reduce stress and enhance rest and relaxation has been abundantly documented. Kundalini yoga massage combines the benefits of yoga and massage and will most definitely improve your overall health and well-being. Although the practice of yoga and massage dates back thousands of years it is unfortunate that many of the ancient techniques are rarely practised. For all intents and purposes, the combination of the techniques outlined in *Kundalini Yoga Massage* are "new." Therefore, it is essential to train more and more practitioners to use the techniques outlined herein. We hope that Kundalini yoga massage will become an integral part of your lifestyle and assist you to achieve optimal health and well-being in all areas of your life.

May you always be blessed with good health.

POSTSCRIPT

PRASHANT JETHALAL

My interest in learning how Eastern philosophies influenced Western minds was kindled because of my mother's deep interest in this subject. As a child I grew up understanding the importance of yoga. When my mother decided to write a book on the subject of yoga I became even more interested in how this ancient practice from the East had so much relevance for the West. In my reading I became aware of how Swami Vivekananda and Nikola Tesla met so long ago and I saw that Vedanta (the essence of Hinduism) and science were not in contradiction with each other but rather in agreement with each other because Vedanta was so scientific. Since their meeting in the nineteenth century scientific developments have been able to demonstrate what the ancient yogis had been saying for centuries.

It is a marvel how ancient yogis with exceptional intellectual skills understood that the nervous system acted as a photographic plate where all our thoughts and impressions were recorded as samskaras on our neural pathways. They were also able to accurately pinpoint that part of the brain called the medulla oblongata controlled the body's regulatory processes of respiration, breath rate, heart rate and digestion. Sitting in the remotest part of the world with no instruments to guide them the yogis made a remarkable discovery that there is a universal, infinite, intelligent force that exists everywhere and in everything including human beings.

Today, modern scientists using sophisticated diagnostic imaging and state-of-the-art telescopes confirm these findings of unity underlying all diversity in the world.[1] We have proof of the neuroplasticity of the brain and we know that there are cohesive, intelligent forces of nature that hold everything together. The discoveries and insights of the ancient yogis are as valid today as they were from the time immemorial simply because they are based on universal truths.

In the early 1890s, Swami Vivekananda was the first spiritual teacher and ambassador to bring yoga and ancient Hindu Vedantic teachings to the West. After Swami Vivekananda successfully delivered his lecture at the World Parliament of Religions in Chicago in 1893 he kindled the interest of several Western scientists, particularly that of Nikola Tesla.

Tesla was a great Western scientist and inventor whilst Swami Vivekananda was a renowned spiritual teacher of Vedic philosophies from the East. While the swami was in America from 1893 onwards he and Tesla had several opportunities to discuss science, yoga and Vedanta. Meeting with Swami Vivekananda greatly stimulated Tesla's interest in Eastern philosophies. Speaking of Tesla, the swami later remarked during a lecture in India, "I myself have been told by some of the best scientific minds of the day how wonderfully rational the conclusions of the Vedanta are. I know of one of them personally who scarcely has time to eat his meal or go out of his laboratory but who would stand by the hour to attend my lectures on the Vedanta; for, as he expresses it, they are so scientific, they

---

1   Dr Norman Doidge, *The Brain that Changes Itself.*

so exactly harmonise with the aspirations of the age and with the conclusions to which modern science is coming at the present time."[2]

Later, in 1895, Vivekananda wrote to an English friend, "Mr. Tesla thinks he can demonstrate mathematically that force and matter are reducible to potential energy. I am to go and see him next week to get this new mathematical demonstration."[3]

Tesla understood the Sanskrit terminology and philosophy and found that it was a good means to describe the physical mechanisms of the universe. Swami Vivekananda was hopeful that Tesla would be able to show that what we call matter is simply potential energy because that would reconcile the teachings of the Vedas with modern science. The swami realised that "in that case, the Vedantic cosmology [would] be placed on the surest of foundations."[4]

Tesla, however, failed to show the identity of energy and matter mathematically. The mathematical proof of the principle didn't come until Albert Einstein published his theory of relativity ($E = MC^2$). What had been known in the East for the last five thousand years was now known to the West.

The Vedas are a collection of ancient scriptures dating back about five thousand years consisting of hymns, prayers, mantras, historical accounting and dissertations on science, literature, politics and the nature of reality. The nature of matter (and anti-matter) and the make-up of the atomic structure are described in the Vedas. Present-day culture in the world may not have been the same had not these two giants in their respective fields met and exchanged their ideas. "A new scientific truth does not triumph by convincing its opponents and making them see the light, but rather because its

2   Swami Vivekananda. Lecture circuit, India.
3   Swami Vivekananda. 1895.
4   Swami Vivekananda. 1895.

opponents eventually die, and a new generation grows up that is familiar with it." – Max Planck[5]

The unique relationship between Nikola Tesla and Swami Vivekananda in the 1890s demonstrated that the foundation of unifying Western science with Eastern wisdom was established a long time ago. The ancient Sanskrit teachings were so exact and so scientific that it completely reconciled and harmonised with modern science. It is because of the pioneering work of Swami Vivekananda and many others that followed the Swami in subsequent decades, that today millions of people throughout the Western world practice yoga and can attest to its benefits.

5   Max Planck, *Scientific Autobiography and Other Papers* (1968).

ABOUT THE AUTHOR

Gita Kalipershad Jethalal was born in Durban, South Africa in the midst of the apartheid regime. During Gita's early childhood the inequality for educational opportunities motivated her family to send her to Dublin, Ireland to complete her college studies. She graduated from the Alexandra Girls' College, a prestigious, all girls private college and completed part of her undergraduate studies at the University College of Dublin.

Upon her return to South Africa she completed her training in radiography at South Africa's largest teaching hospital, King Edward the VIII. From 1974 to 1987 she worked in several hospitals in South Africa and gained invaluable experience in dealing with human suffering.

She came from a deeply spiritual family steeped in doing humanitarian work. During the early 1960s and 1970s there was a large influx of spiritual leaders from India setting up ashrams in and around Durban. Since her family resided in close proximity to the Ramakrishna Centre and the Divine Life Society she was exposed to yoga from a very young age. From early childhood Gita's thinking was greatly influenced by the profound teachings of Swami Vivekananda and Swami Paramahansa Yogananda, renowned author of *Autobiography of a Yogi*. Gita got married in 1980, and in 1987, together with her husband and son, she immigrated to Canada to get away from the unstable and unsafe conditions in South Africa.

In Canada, she decided to pursue her lifelong goal of becoming a chiropractor and enrolled at the Canadian Memorial Chiropractic College as a full-time student.

After graduating in 1991 Dr Gita started her own private practice. Since 1991 she has been owner and clinic director of a multidisciplinary rehabilitation clinic in Toronto. In 1992, Dr Gita met Swami Jyotirmayananda who is the living embodiment of truth, peace, bliss and humility. She was so impressed with Swamiji's wealth of timeless wisdom and his great command of spiritual knowledge of yoga and Vedanta that she immediately became a member of the Yoga Research Foundation. Dr Gita continues to practice integral yoga as taught by Swami Jyotirmayananda together with the knowledge acquired from other masters and incorporates their combined teachings into all aspects of her life. Integral yoga is a way of life and thought that synthesises the various aspects of ancient yoga traditions into a comprehensive plan of personality integration. Over the past twenty-four years she has treated thousands of patients with a variety of musculo-skeletal disorders. Dr Gita has always adopted a multidisciplinary approach to treating patients.

Being in the health care field for the last forty years Dr Gita has gained extensive experience in treating stress-related musculo-skeletal disorders. Having seen the positive impact on patients being treated with Kundalini yoga massage, in addition to traditional therapies, Dr Gita wanted to share this knowledge so that others can benefit. It was with this goal in mind that she decided to write this book. Kundalini yoga massage focuses on a series of techniques to activate the seven chakras by removing physiological blockages and thereby enhancing the flow of prana (vital energy).

In this book, Dr Gita has combined her decades of knowledge of Western science with her lifetime of self-acquired knowledge of yoga and the wisdom of Eastern philosophies to show the powerful link between Western modalities, yoga and Kundalini yoga massage in healing. Dr Gita is a strong proponent of self-knowledge and self-realisation. Philosopher Kahlil Gibran put it succinctly when he said that self-knowledge is "[1]as the sea: boundless and measureless," as knowledge acquired by the self transcends all limiting boundaries.

Today, Dr Gita lives with her husband and son in Toronto. She is looking forward to using her knowledge and expertise to assist and uplift those with pain and suffering, especially in developing countries.

To show her gratitude to Swamiji for his teachings and guidance over the years and to give back to those who are in need, Dr Gita will be donating a percentage of the proceeds from the sale of this book to Swamiji at the Yoga Research Foundation in Miami and to the Lalita Jyoti Anathalaya Orphanage and School for Girls in Bihar, India.

---

1   Kahlil Gibran, *The Prophet* 1923

SAMPLE FORMS
FOR PROFESSIONAL
THERAPISTS

PATIENT CONSENT FORMS

<u>CONSENT FORM</u>

I hereby request and consent to the performance and application of:

☐ Yoga Massage Therapy

and other procedures, including various modes of physical therapy and, if necessary prescribed and/or supervised exercise therapy and massage therapy. I understand that I am authorizing the therapist and/or any registered practitioner working in the clinic.

I have had the opportunity to discuss with the therapist and/or with other office/clinic personnel, the nature and purpose of all procedures. I understand that the results are not guaranteed.

I further understand and am informed that as in all areas of health care, as well as rehabilitation exercise there are some risks to treatment. I wish to rely on the therapist to exercise judgment during the course of the procedure, based upon the facts then known, that are in my best interests.

I, _____ have read the above mentioned and I have also had the opportunity to ask questions about this consent and by signing below I agree to the above mentioned procedures. I intend to this consent form to cover the entire course of all my treatments.

_____   _____

Patient Signature   Date

PATIENT HISTORY FORM
AND PROGRESS NOTES

YOGA MASSAGE HEALTH HISTORY FORM

FYI: It is essential to provide accurate health history as this ensures that you to receive a professional massage treatment, and this assists the therapist to provide a proper treatment plan. If your health status changes in the future please let the therapist know. All information gathered is confidential. Your written authorization is legally required before any of this information can be released.

Personal Information:

Name: _____ Date: _____ ☐ Male ☐ Female
     (FIRST)   (LAST)   (DD/MM/YY)
Date of Birth: _____ Height: _____ Weight: _____ Occupation: _____
    (DD/MM/YY)
Address: _____ City: _____ Postal Code: _____
Home Phone: (_____) _____-_____ Work Phone: (_____) _____-_____
Doctor: _____ Phone: (_____) _____-_____ May I contact? ☐ Yes ☐ No
Emergency Contact Name: _____ Phone: (_____) _____-_____

Have you had massage before? ☐ Yes ☐ No If Yes, was it for relaxation or other reason:
Current Medications: _____
Previous Major Illnesses or Operation/s: _____
Accidents (Specify Dates): _____ Fractures: _____
Other Medical condition/s (e.g.: cardiac conditions): _____
Family history (major illnesses or operations): _____

What is your major symptom/problem? _____	**HAVE YOU HAD ANY:**	**Date:**
When did your symptoms begin? _____	Automobile accidents?	_____
Have you had this problem before? _____	Surgeries?	_____
Is your condition getting progressively worse? Yes ☐ No ☐	Broken bones?	_____
Is this problem: ☐ Constant ☐ Comes and goes	Falls/Head injuries?	_____

How does it feel? ☐ Burning ☐ Sharp ☐ Shooting ☐ Dull
    ☐ Aching ☐ Stiff ☐ Tingling ☐ Throbbing   **STRESSORS:**
    ☐ Swelling ☐ Other_____   ☐ Smoking Packs/Day: _____
Circle below the severity of your pain on a scale of 0 to 10:   ☐ Alcohol Drinks/Week: _____
(No Pain) 0 1 2 3 4 5 6 7 8 9 10 (Severe Pain)   ☐ Coffee/Caffeine Drinks Cup/Day: ____
What makes your condition better? _____   ☐ High Stress Level **Reason:** _____
What makes your condition worse? _____
Does it interfere with your: ☐ Work ☐ Sleep ☐ Daily Routine ☐ Recreation

Please indicate all conditions you have experienced. Mark "C" for CURRENT or "P" for PAST:

Joint/Soft Tissue Discomfort:
__ Arms
__ Upper Back
__ Mid Back
__ Lower Back
__ Degenerative Discs
__ Feet
__ Hands
__ Hips
__ Jaw
__ Knees
__ Legs
__ Neck
__ Osteo Arthritis
__ Rheumatiod
__ Sciatica Limitation of Movement
__ Shoulders
__ Other: _____

Skin:
__ Rashes
__ Itching
__ Bruise Easily
__ Dryness
__ Boils
__ Other: _____

General Symptoms:
__ Fainting
__ Dizziness
__ Loss of Sleep
__ Fatigue
__ Nervousness
__ Sudden Weight Loss/Gain
__ Numbness
__ Tingling
__ Paralysis
__ Headaches

Cardiovascular:
__ High Blood Pressure
__ Low Blood Pressure
__ Coronary Disease
__ Heart Attack
__ Phlebitis
__ Stroke/CVA
__ Pacemaker
__ Hear Murmur
__ Palpitations
__ Varicose Veins
__ Poor Circulation
__ Swelling of the Ankles

Infectious:
__ Hepatitis
__ Tuberculosis
__ HIV
__ Herpes
__ Cold
__ Flu
__ Athlete's Foot
__ Warts
__ Other: _____

Digestive:
__ Poor Appetite
__ Belching/Gas
__ Constipation
__ Diarrhea
__ Nausea
__ Ulcer
__ Vomiting

Eye, Ear, Nose & Throat:
__ Allergies
__ Frequent Colds
__ Glasses or Contacts
__ Hearing Aid

__ Hearing Loss
__ Sinus Infection
__ Swollen Glands

FEMALES: Are you pregnant? ☐ Yes ☐ No

Please indicate all conditions you have experienced. Mark "C" for CURRENT and "P" for PAST:

Reproductive:
__ Pregnant
__ Due Date: _____
__ Painful Menstruation
__ Heavy Flow
__ Irregular Cycle
__ Swollen Breasts
__ Menopausal

__ Pre-Menopausal
__ Post-Menopausal
__ Birth Control
__ Type: _____

Respiratory:
__ Chronic Cough
__ Bronchitis
__ Asthma
__ Hay Fever
__ Difficulty Breathing
__ Smoking
__ Emphysema
__ Pneumonia

Activities/movements that is painful to perform:
☐ Sitting ☐ Standing ☐ Walking ☐ Bending ☐ Lying Down ☐ Driving ☐ Reading ☐ Getting Up
List any medications you are taking: _____

Lifestyle Questions:
Regular eating habits: ☐ Yes ☐ No
Do you take Vitamins? ☐ Yes ☐ No
Type: _____
Frequency: _____
Regular Exercise: ☐ Yes ☐ No
Type: _____
Frequency: _____

Energy Level: ☐ High ☐ Average ☐ Low
   Do you suffer from stress? ☐ Yes ☐ No
Type: _____
Do you use a computer? ☐ Yes ☐ No
   How many hours per day? _____

Please read carefully and sign:
I attest that the information I have provided are true and complete to the best of my knowledge.
I understand the information I have provided on this form is confidential and will not be released without my written consent.
I consent to yoga massage treatments by the below named massage therapist.
I also understand that I am responsible for any charges incurred in the course of my treatment.
I understand that 24-hour notice is required to reschedule all future appointments, or full charges will apply.

_____
Patient Name (Please PRINT)

_____
Patient Signature

_____
Date (DD/MM/YY)

For Massage Therapist ONLY:

FRONT   BACK
Circle any focal areas

Treat Therapist: _____
Duration of Massage: _____ Cost: _____
Techniques used: _____
_____

Comments: _____

Self Care Recommendations: _____
_____
_____
_____

PATIENT FEEDBACK FORM

FEEDBACK FORM

Either Tick "✓" or Circle the correct answer
Explanation is required for Question 15 and 17

1. Did the therapist introduce himself/herself and address you by your name?

   Yes____   No____

2. Did the therapist explain what they were going to do before you started your treatment? (eg. Instructions on disrobing and where to keep your valuables whilst having the massage).

   Yes____   No____

3. Did the therapist explain all the areas he or she was going to massage?

   Yes____   No____   A little bit _____

4. Did the therapist ensure that you were comfortable during the treatment?

   Yes____   No____

5. Did the therapist go over the health form with you and address your health concerns? Yes____   No____

6. Was the therapist talkative? Too Much____   A little____   Mostly Silent____

7. Did the therapist explain all 7 Steps of the massage technique in Yoga Massage?

   Yes____   No____

8. Judging from the pace, did the therapist appear to be in a hurry?

   Yes____   No____

9. Did you notice a consistent flow during the massage?

   Most of the time____   Some of the time____   Not at all____

10. On a scale of 1-10 how would you rate the therapist? (0 being very bad and 10 being excellent)

    0   1   2   3   4   5   6   7   8   9   10

11. Evaluate the effectiveness of the massage (0 very bad and 10 being excellent)

    0   1   2   3   4   5   6   7   8   9   10

12. Did the therapist spend too much or not enough time in any particular area?

Yes_____ No_____

13. Did the therapist explain the possible side-effects from receiving a massage: Soreness, Dizziness, Flu-like symptoms, Dehydration, Headache, Bruising, and temporary increase in pain?

Yes_____ No____

14. Did the therapist ask you to drink extra water and explain the reason why you have to?

Yes_____ No_____

15. If you ever received a professional massage before: what did you like or dislike compared to your other massages?

Explain:_____

_____

_____

_____

16. Did the therapist explain why it is necessary for you to receive more massages in the near future?

Yes_____ No_____

17. Any other comments?

_____

_____

_____

DYSFUNCTION IN FOOT MECHANICS CAUSES DYSFUNCTION IN BODY MECHANICS AND AFFECTS THE FLOW OF PRANA (LIFE FORCE)

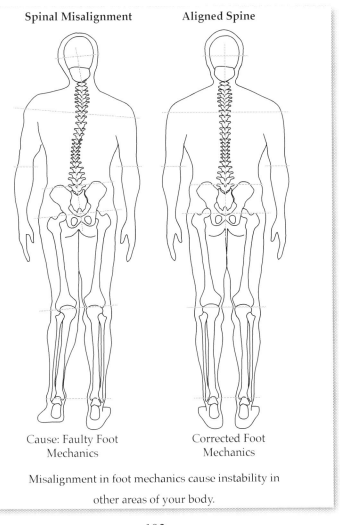

Spinal Misalignment   Aligned Spine

Cause: Faulty Foot Mechanics   Corrected Foot Mechanics

Misalignment in foot mechanics cause instability in other areas of your body.

BIOMECHANICAL ASSESSMENT FORM

BIOMECHANCIAL
ASSESSMENT

Name: Date:

Chief Complaint:

Weight Bearing Examination

- Forefoot to Rearfoot Relationship

Right   Rearfoot

FOREFOOT	Varus	Perpendicular	Valgus
Varus	Cavoid	2	3
Perpendicular	4	Neutral	8
Valgus	7	8	Planus

Left   Rearfoot

FOREFOOT	Varus	Perpendicular	Valgus
Varus	Cavoid	2	3
Perpendicular	4	Neutral	8
Valgus	7	8	Planus

Left Foot: varus   Right foot: varus

- Clacaneus to Tibia Relationship

	Right Calcaneus	Left Calcaneus
Inverted		
Perpendicular		
Everted	*	*

Range of motion

Joints	MPJ	Ankle	STJ	MTJ	IPJ
ALL NORMAL					

Foot type: pes planus

GAIT ANALYSIS FORM

GAIT
ANALYSIS

Stance Phase		
Excessive medial longitudinal arch drop RIGHT LEFT	Tibial varum	Haglunds deformity RIGHT LEFT
Excessive medial long arch height RIGHT LEFT	Tibial valgum	Range of motion
Talar head prominence RIGHT LEFT	Genu varum	Tight hamstrings RIGHT LEFT
Prominent 1st metatarsal head RIGHT LEFT	Genu recurvatum	Kyphosis
Prominent 5th metatarsal head RIGHT LEFT	Genu valgum	Scoliosis
Forefoot splay RIGHT LEFT	Excessive external tibial rotation	Plantar lesions
Foot shape CONCAVE CONVEX RF LF	Excessive internal tibial rotation	Other

Gait Phase		
Ataxic	Asymptomatic	Apropulsive
Leg length discrepancy LEFT LEG _____CM RIGHT LEG _____CM	Shoulder tilt TOWRARDS RIGHT TOWARDS LEFT	Excessive arm swing RIGHT LEFT

DX - Diagnosis   see prescription

Treatment:
Daily use of orthotics to control the amount of subtalar join pronation reduces the amount of upper and lower leg rotation thereby alleviating lower back strain; hallux deviation; increases meta tarsal phalangeal joint (MTPJ) range of motion (ROM).

BIBLIOGRAPHY

Sivanada Yoga Vedanta Centre. *Yoga Mind & Body*. Firefly Canada, 1996.

His Holiness Maharishi Mahesh Yogi. *The Science of Being and the Art of Living*. Penguin Gray, January 1995.

Simmha, Anton. *Ashtanga Yoga*. Raincoast Books, 2003.

Brown, Barbara D. *New Body, New Mind*. Bantam Books, July 1974.

Chopra, Dr Deepak, *The Seven Spiritual Laws of Success*, Amber Allen Publishing and New World Library 1994

Monks of the Ramakrishna Order. *Meditation*. Ramakrishna Vedanta Centre, 1972.

Maltz, Maxwell. *Psycho Cybernetics*. Wilshire Book Company and Prentice Hall Inc., 2001.

Paramahansa Yogananda, Swami. *Autobiography of a Yogi*. Self Realization Fellowship, 1973.

Paramahansa Yogananda, Swami. *Journey to Self-Realization*. Self Realization Fellowship, 1997.

Paramahansa, Yogananda, Swami *Scientific Healing Affirmation, 1981*

Dharam Vir Mangala. *Kundalini and Kriya Yoga*. Winsome Books India, 2003.

Zukav, Gary. *The Seat of the Soul*. Free Press, 1989.

Journal of Hindu Dharma Review (Canadian Council of Hindus) 7, no. 3 (1993).

Swananda, Swami. *Raja Yoga*. Translated by Swami Vivekananda. 1990.

Jyotirmayananda, Swami. *International Yoga Guide* 50, no. 9 (May 2013).

Jyotirmayananda, Swami. *International Yoga Guide* 47, no. 11 (July 2010).

Jyotirmayananda, Swami. *International Yoga Guide* 47, no. 12 (August 2010).

Jyotirmayananda, Swami. *International Yoga Guide* 46, no. 1 (September2008).

Jyotirmayananda, Swami. *International Yoga Guide* 48, no. 2 (October 2008).

Jyotirmayananda, Swami. *International Yoga Guide* 50, no. 2 (October 2012).

Jyotirmayananda, Swami. *International Yoga Guide* 46, no. 11 (July 2009).

Jyotirmayananda, Swami. *International Yoga Guide* 49, no. 5 (July 2012).

Jyotirmayananda, Swami. *International Yoga Guide* 49, no. 3 (November 2011).

Jyotirmayananda, Swami. *International Yoga Guide* 46, no. 6 (February 2011).

Jyotirmayananda, Swami. *International Yoga Guide* 48 (January 2011).

Jyotirmayananda, Swami. *Concentration and Meditation*. International Yoga Society, 2013.

Sivananda, Sri Swami. Divine Life Society of South Africa.

Guidelines from Massage Therapy Association of Ontario, 1991.

Jyotirmayananda, Swami. *Yoga Secrets of Psychic Power*. Swami Lalitananada International Yoga Society, Miami, Florida, 1974.

Vivekananda, Swami. Introduction to *The Yoga Sutras of Patanjali*, by Sage Patanjali. Duncan Baird Publishers, 2007.

Vivekananda, Swami. *Powers of the Mind*. Sri Gouranga Press Private Limited, Eighth Impression, March 1973.

Wikipedia Free Encyclopaedia Online for a variety of definitions.

Benson, Dr Herbert. Mind-Body Medical Institute, University of Harvard.

Tolle, Eckhart. *The Power of Now*. Namaste Publishing Inc., 1997.

Tolle, Eckhart. *A New Earth: Awakening to your Life's Purpose*. Penguin Group, 2005.

Murphy, Dr. Joseph, The Power of Your Subconscious Mind. Prentice Hall Inc., 1983.

Doidge, Dr Norman. *The Brain that Changes Itself*. Penguin Books, 2007.

Newberg, Dr Andrew. *The Mystical Mind*. Fortress Press, 1999.

Rhadakrishnan, Dr Sarvepalli. *East and West: Some Reflections*. New York: Harper and Brothers, 1953.

Newburg, Dr. Andrew. *andrewnewburg.com. "How do meditation and prayer change our brains?"*

Printed in the United States
By Bookmasters